Physical Assessment and History Taking:

An Easy Guide for Healthcare Professionals

M.A Gorre

Contents

Preface

The Unseen Foundations of Healthcare: An In-Depth Exploration into Physical Examination and History-Taking
In the rapidly evolving world of healthcare, amidst the maze of complex diagnostic tools and medical procedures, lies the cornerstone of patient care—Physical Examination and History Taking. It's tempting to think that in a world awash with digital technology and precision diagnostics, the fundamental acts of listening, questioning, and tactile examination may have lost their lustre. Yet, the reality is far from it. The role of these basic techniques has only become more significant as they remain irreplaceable in providing insights into a patient's condition that are both deep and nuanced.

The Quintessential Art of Medicine

Physical examination and history-taking serve as clinical tools and an essential part of the art of medicine. They are the mediums through which a healthcare provider can connect with a patient, build trust, and gather vital information to inform all subsequent stages of care. Despite our technological advancements, machines still cannot interpret the look in a patient's eyes or detect the nuances in their voice when they describe their symptoms. Nor can they experience that intuitive feeling a seasoned physician gets when something feels "off" during a physical examination. These subtle but invaluable cues can often be the missing pieces of a complex medical puzzle.

Why This Book Is Essential Now

We're in an era where machine learning algorithms, telemedicine consultations, and robotic surgeries increasingly guide diagnostics and treatment modalities. While these developments have significantly improved aspects of patient care, they also risk overshadowing the foundational skills of history-taking and physical examination. We wrote this book to shine a light on these cornerstones, to reveal how they could and should seamlessly integrate with modern practices, providing a more comprehensive, humane approach to patient care.

Target Audience and the Reach Beyond

Who Should Read This Book?

This tome aims to serve a wide variety of readers:

- **Medical Students**: In your formative years, this book can serve as a cornerstone text, laying the foundation for your medical knowledge to grow.

- **Nursing Students**: Given your critical role in patient care, the skills outlined here directly apply to your daily responsibilities.

- **Healthcare Practitioners**: Whether you're a general physician, a specialist, or a nurse with decades of experience, consider this book a refresher course that can bring new insights into your established routine.

- **Medical Educators**: Those responsible for shaping the future generations of healthcare providers will find theory and practical exercises to integrate into their curriculum.

- **Interested Laypersons**: While this book is technical, the importance of the subject matter transcends the medical community. It provides valuable insights into how healthcare providers think and make decisions.

How to Navigate Through the Book

- **Comprehensive Study**: For beginners, especially students, we recommend a sequential reading from start to finish, accompanied by practical exercises presented at the end of each chapter.

- **As a Reference Manual**: Experienced professionals can use this book as a comprehensive reference, navigating directly to topics or sections that address their immediate needs or questions.

- **Interactive Learning**: Case studies, questionnaires, and interactive exercises are peppered throughout the book, allowing for a more engaged reading experience. These are useful for both novices and experts.

- **Appendices and Resources**: Extensive appendices offer quick-reference guides, cheat sheets, and additional resources for further exploration. They are designed to be practical and handy during real clinical work.

- **Further Learning**: Each chapter concludes with an annotated list of other readings, academic papers, and additional resources curated to guide those interested in diving deeper into the minutiae of each topic.

Embarking on a Journey of Lifelong Learning

What lies ahead is not merely a series of chapters to be read but a journey through the rich tapestry of medical practice. This book, replete with evidence-based insights, real-world anecdotes, and actionable advice, aims to instill a keen understanding and deep appreciation for the art and science of physical examination and history taking.

So, open the first page and step into a world where the past and the present of medicine coalesce, offering you the skills and knowledge to survive and thrive in the ever-changing landscape of healthcare.

Welcome to your indispensable guide to mastering the very soul of medicine.

Introduction

Tracing the Arc of Time: The History and Evolution of Physical Examination and History Taking

As you crack open this book and embark on a quest to master the fundamentals of healthcare, it's worth pausing to appreciate the roots of the practices we're about to delve into. Physical examination and history taking aren't just rituals conducted in hospitals and clinics worldwide; they are time-honored techniques that have evolved over millennia, intertwined with the very history of medicine itself.

The Dawn of an Era: Ancient Civilizations

Long before the invention of X-rays, MRI machines, and blood tests, ancient civilizations like the Egyptians, Greeks, and Chinese were already employing rudimentary forms of physical examination and history taking. Whether it was the palpation of the abdomen, inspection of the skin, or simple observations of a patient's demeanor, these early medical practitioners understood the power of direct human observation and interaction.

The Medieval and Renaissance Developments

Fast forward to the medieval period, where figures like Avicenna—known as the "Father of Modern Medicine"—compiled medical encyclopedias that emphasized the importance of history taking in the diagnosis and treatment of diseases. By the time the Renaissance arrived, anatomical dissections became a cornerstone of medical understanding, further deepening the role of physical examination.

The Age of Enlightenment to the Modern Era

The Enlightenment and the centuries that followed brought a more systematic approach to these practices. The invention of the stethoscope by René Laennec in 1816 revolutionized the field, offering a more precise way to study the human body. Fast forward to the 20th and 21st centuries, and we find that despite exponential advancements in technology, the basics of laying hands and eyes on the patient, and asking the right questions, remain irreplaceable.

The Pillars of Modern Healthcare: Diagnostic and Therapeutic Roles

Diagnostic Role: The First Step in a Medical Journey

When a patient walks into a healthcare setting, the first and perhaps most crucial step is an accurate diagnosis. Here, history taking acts as the map, laying out the contours of the patient's symptoms, lifestyle, and previous medical history. Physical examination then acts as the compass, guiding the clinician toward what needs closer inspection.

Together, they offer the initial set of clues that inform which path of investigation to take.

Therapeutic Role: Beyond Diagnosis

Less appreciated but equally important is the therapeutic role of physical examination and history taking. The act of being heard and examined can be comforting to a patient, offering psychological relief that's a form of therapy in itself. Moreover, the insights gained from these initial steps often shape the entire course of treatment, from the choice of medication to the need for surgery or other interventions.

Intersecting with Modern Medicine

In today's world of targeted therapies, gene editing, and telemedicine, one might wonder how these ancient arts fit in. The answer is: seamlessly. Even the most advanced predictive algorithms or diagnostic tests require the rich context that only a thorough history and examination can provide. They help narrow down the scope of possibilities, informing more specialized tests and treatment options, and as such, they remain the indispensable first steps in the increasingly complex dance of modern medicine.

As we turn the page to delve into the nitty-gritty of how to master these essential skills, keep in mind that you're participating in a lineage that stretches back thousands of years. You're not just learning techniques; you're becoming a part of an ancient, noble tradition dedicated to understanding and alleviating the suffering of human beings. Welcome to the enthralling world of physical examination and history taking, the twin pillars upon which the colossal edifice of healthcare stands.

Chapter One

The Importance of Medical History

P rinciples and Preparation

Introduction

As the first step in the diagnostic process, taking a patient's medical history is often likened to unlocking a treasure chest of clinical information. A thorough history provides clues to the patient's immediate concern and enlightens the healthcare provider about the patient's past and ongoing medical issues, lifestyle, and even emotional well-being. This chapter aims to elucidate why this seemingly straightforward practice is critically important and how to conduct it effectively.

Objectives:

- Understand the significance of a thorough medical history in patient care.

- Learn how to collect a patient's medical history systematical-ly.

- Grasp the nuances of asking the right questions and listening actively

Topics Covered:

Why Medical History Matters

- The gateway to diagnosis: how a good history often solves half the puzzle

- Risk stratification: identifying patients who need immediate attention versus those who don't

- Chronology of illness: tracing the sequence of events that led to the current state

The Structure of Medical History

- Chief Complaint (CC)

- History of Present Illness (HPI)

- Past Medical History (PMH)

- Family History

- Social History

- Review of Systems (ROS)

The Skill of Questioning

- Open-ended vs. closed-ended questions

- Adapting your language to the patient's understanding

- Overcoming barriers such as language or cultural differences

Active Listening

- How to listen for what's unsaid as much as what's said

- Picking up on verbal and non-verbal cues

- Confirming and clarifying information

Case Studies:

The Silent Clue

- Listening attentively during history taking revealed a vital clue leading to a rare diagnosis.

Lost in Translation

- I was managing a case where language barriers almost led to a medical error and how to avoid it.

Self-Assessment:

- Quiz on the components of medical history

- Interactive scenario: Taking history from a standardized patient

- Checklist for effective questioning and listening

Self-Assessment: Test Your Skills

Are you ready to put your knowledge to the test and further hone your skills in medical history taking? This interactive self-assessment section is designed to help you reinforce what you've learned and build your confidence as a healthcare professional. Here's what you'll find:

1. Quiz on the Components of Medical History:

- Challenge your understanding of medical history by taking a comprehensive quiz. Test your knowledge of critical components, including identifying data, chief complaints, past medical history, family history, and more. Each question is designed to reinforce your grasp of these crucial elements.

2. Interactive Scenario: Taking History from a Standardized Patient:

- Step into the shoes of a healthcare provider and engage in a realistic scenario. Interact with a standardized patient to practice the art of history-taking in a controlled environment. Navigate through various patient procedures designed to help you apply your skills and refine your approach.

3. Checklist for Effective Questioning and Listening:
- A valuable tool for every healthcare professional, this checklist provides a structured framework for conducting compelling patient interviews. Ensure you're asking the right questions, actively listening to your patients, and gathering the essential information for accurate assessments.

This self-assessment section is an integral part of your journey to becoming a proficient and compassionate healthcare provider. Use it to reinforce your learning, fine-tune your skills, and gain the confidence you need to excel in your clinical practice. Whether you're a student or an experienced practitioner, these self-assessment tools will help you achieve excellence in medical history taking.

Ready to challenge yourself and take your skills to the next level? Dive into these interactive assessments and see your knowledge and competence grow. Your patients will thank you for it!

This description highlights the interactive and educational nature of the self-assessment section in your book, encouraging readers to actively engage with the content and improve their medical history-taking skills.

Summary

As we delve deeper into the art and science of physical examination and history taking, it becomes evident that these practices are not merely procedural but demand skill, empathy, and attention to detail that separates an average healthcare provider from an excellent one. And it all starts with taking a solid, comprehensive medical history. In the subsequent chapters, we will build upon this foundation, focusing on the physical examination and other aspects that complete the diagnostic cycle.

Chapter Two

Significance in Diagnosis

The importance of medical history in diagnosis cannot be overstated. Medical circles often say that a thorough history will provide enough information to diagnose up to 80% of conditions without further tests or examinations. While this figure might vary depending on the context, the essential idea remains: a comprehensive history offers invaluable diagnostic clues.

When a patient presents with a set of symptoms, the history aids in differentiating between various possible conditions that might give similarly. For example, chest pain could indicate cardiac issues, gastrointestinal problems, or even anxiety. A detailed history will include questions about the nature of the pain, its duration, any triggering factors, and associated symptoms, thus helping to narrow down the list of potential diagnoses.

Furthermore, medical history brings to light preexisting conditions, medications, and familial tendencies, all significant in risk stratification. It helps clinicians decide who needs immediate, aggressive treatment and who can be managed conservatively.

How It Informs the Physical Exam

Medical history serves as a roadmap for the physical examination that follows. The physical exam can feel like navigating a labyrinth in the dark without a clear record. On the other hand, when you know what you're looking for, you can conduct a targeted, adequate examination.

For instance, if a patient's history indicates episodes of breathlessness and nocturnal cough, the clinician will focus on a detailed respiratory and cardiovascular examination, potentially saving valuable time in diagnosis and treatment. Similarly, a history of recent travel to tropical regions would prompt an exhaustive look for signs of infectious diseases that are prevalent in those areas.

Moreover, specific findings in the history can indicate the need for specialized tests. If a patient reports severe, episodic headaches accompanied by visual disturbances, it will prompt the clinician to perhaps initiate imaging studies or neurological tests in addition to a physical examination.

Lastly, the medical history also impacts the sequence and approach of the physical exam. For example, if a patient reports severe abdominal pain, that area might be examined last to minimize discomfort, or unique positioning might facilitate the examination.

In summary, medical history plays a pivotal role in making an accurate diagnosis and guides the healthcare provider in conducting a targeted and effective physical examination. Together, they create a synergistic effect that enhances patient care, making each an indispensable part of the diagnostic process.

Chapter Three

Setting Up for Success

Introduction

The physical and emotional atmosphere in which a medical examination occurs dramatically influences the quality of care provided. A thoughtfully prepared space can increase the accuracy of a diagnosis, enhance patient comfort, and facilitate clear and open communication between healthcare providers and patients.

Environment Preparation

Physical Setting

- **The value of a clean, organized space:** A neat and orderly examination room minimizes distractions, allows more efficient use of time and can reduce medical errors. It also fosters a sense of professionalism that can put the patient at ease.

- **Appropriate lighting and its impact on examination:** Good lighting is essential for many aspects of a physical exam, from evaluating skin tone and condition to conducting a thorough eye examination. LED lights with adjustable brightness can be a good option.

- **Comfort factors:** Ergonomic chairs and adjustable examination tables make the process smoother for the healthcare provider and the patient. Consider temperature controls and noise reduction features to create a comfortable environment.

Psychological Factors

- **Creating a space that encourages open dialogue:** A private, quiet room will make the patient feel safe and more willing to share sensitive information, which is crucial for an accurate history and diagnosis.

- **Privacy considerations:** The room should have curtains or blinds and a lockable door to ensure patient privacy during potentially vulnerable moments.

- **Patient comfort:** A comfortable patient is a more communicative patient. Having tissues, water, and clear step-by-step instructions can make a significant difference.

Necessary Tools and Instruments

General Tools

- **Examination Table:** An adjustable table covered with disposable paper for hygiene.

- **Stethoscope:** For auscultation of heart and lung sounds.

- **Blood Pressure Cuff (Sphygmomanometer):** To check the patient's blood pressure.

- **Thermometer:** For measuring body temperature.

- **Penlight:** Useful for eye examinations and to observe pupillary response.

- **Tongue Depressors:** For oral examinations.

Specialty Tools

- **Otoscope:** For examining the inner ear.

- **Ophthalmoscope:** To examine the back of the eye, including the retina.

- **Reflex Hammer:** For neurological evaluations of reflexes.

- **Spirometer:** To assess lung function in cases of suspected respiratory issues.

- **Electrocardiogram (ECG) Machine:** For monitoring heart

activity.

Hygiene and Safety

- **Hand Hygiene:** Wash hands thoroughly before and after each examination. Alcohol-based sanitizers can also be effective.

- **Personal Protective Equipment (PPE):** Wear gloves during the examination and a mask if respiratory issues are suspected or during pandemics.

- **Sterilization:** All reusable instruments must be sterilized between uses.

- **Disposal:** In medical waste bins, single-use items like tongue depressors should be appropriately disposed of.

This thorough preparation and setup are not merely ancillary to the examination process but integral to it. A well-prepared healthcare provider is better equipped to diagnose and treat patients effectively, elevating the standard of care provided.

Chapter Four

Professionalism and Ethics

Introduction

In medical practice, professionalism and ethics are not merely supplementary; they are integral to providing quality care. This chapter will explore the fundamental principles underpinning medical ethics, focusing on informed consent and maintaining patient privacy and confidentiality.

Objectives

- Understand the importance of professionalism and ethics in healthcare.

- Learn the principles of informed consent and how to obtain it.

- Recognize the legal and ethical obligations related to patient privacy and confidentiality.

Topics Covered:

Professionalism

- **Definition and Importance:** Professionalism refers to the conduct, aims, or qualities that characterize a profession or professional person. In healthcare, this includes everything from how you dress to how you interact with patients and colleagues. The importance of professionalism extends beyond first impressions; it sets the tone for the entire patient-provider relationship and the quality of care delivered.

Ethics

- **Code of Ethics:** Most healthcare providers operate under a code of ethics that outlines their responsibilities, including honesty, integrity, and patient advocacy. Understanding and adhering to these principles is essential for building trust and providing adequate care.

Informed Consent

- **Principles:** Informed consent is the process by which a healthcare provider informs a patient about the available op-

tions for treatment, including the potential risks and benefits, so the patient can make an educated decision about their
care.

- **How to Obtain:** The healthcare provider should use clear
  and simple language to ensure the patient fully understands
  the implications of their choices. Consent forms are generally used, and the patient should sign thesestraightforward.

Patient Privacy and Confidentiality

- **Legal Framework:** Laws like the Health Insurance Portability and Accountability Act (HIPAA) in the U.S. outline
  healthcare providers' obligationsExaminin to protect patient
  information.

- **Practical Measures:** This includes everything from secure
  storage of medical records to ensuring patient confidentiality
  during consultations. Always consider the patient's privacy
  when discussing their case or medical history, whether in
  verbal conversations or electronic communications.

Case Studies:

Case 1: A Breach of Confidentiality

- An examination of the consequences when a healthcare
  provider discusses a patient's medical condition with a col-

league in a public setting, leads to a breach of patient confidentiality.

Case 2: Informed Consent Gone Wrong

- An analysis of a situation where a patient was not fully informed about the risks of a medical procedure, leading to ethical and legal complications.

Self-Assessment:

- Questions on the fundamental principles of medical ethics

- Multiple-choice quiz on the steps for obtaining informed consent

- Scenario-based questions on maintaining patient confidentiality

Self-Assessment: Test Your Ethical Knowledge

1. Key Principles of Medical Ethics:

Question 1: Which of the following principles of medical ethics emphasizes the obligation to "not harm"?

A) Autonomy

B) Beneficence

C) Non-maleficence

D) Justice

Answer: C) Non-maleficence

Question 2: What does "autonomy" refer to in medical ethics?

A) The obligation to provide benefits to patients

B) The right of patients to make their own decisions regarding their medical care

C) The fair distribution of healthcare resources

D) The duty to be truthful with patients

Answer: B) The right of patients to make their own decisions regarding their medical care

2. Obtaining Informed Consent:

Question 3: What is NOT a critical step in obtaining informed consent?

A) Providing information about the proposed treatment or procedure

B) Ensuring the patient fully understands the information provided

C) Coercing the patient into accepting the treatment

D) Allowing the patient to ask questions and seek clarification

Answer: C) Coercing the patient into accepting the treatment

Question 4: True or False: Informed consent is a one-time process and does not need to be revisited if the patient's condition or treatment plan changes.

Answer: False. Informed consent should be an ongoing process and may need to be revisited if there are changes in the patient's condition or treatment plan.

3. Maintaining Patient Confidentiality:

Question 5: What is the primary ethical reason for maintaining patient confidentiality?

A) To protect the reputation of the healthcare provider

B) To ensure that patients feel comfortable sharing sensitive information

C) To avoid legal consequences

D) To minimize paperwork and administrative burdens

Answer: B) To ensure that patients feel comfortable sharing sensitive information

Question 6: In which of the following situations is it acceptable to disclose a patient's confidential information without their consent?

A) When discussing the case with colleagues during a lunch break

B) When a family member calls and requests information about the patient's condition

C) When required by law or for public health reasons

D) Never, unless the patient gives explicit consent

Answer: C) When required by law or for public health reasons

These self-assessment questions and answers can help readers reinforce their understanding of medical ethics, informed consent, and patient confidentiality while ensuring they follow ethical principles in their healthcare practice.

Summary

The principles of professionalism and ethics are foundational to medical practice. They establish trust, ensure quality, and uphold the rights and dignity of the patient. As a healthcare provider, your commitment to these principles is not just a requirement but a pledge to maintain the highest standards of medical care.

Chapter Five

Initial Patient Interaction

Introduction

The first interaction between a healthcare provider and a patient sets the tone for the entire relationship. From building rapport to effective communication, the initial meeting is an opportunity to establish trust and lay the groundwork for successful healthcare outcomes. This chapter will focus on strategies and best practices for an impactful initial patient interaction.

Objectives

- Understand the importance of the initial patient interaction in establishing a trusting relationship.

- Learn practical techniques for building rapport with patients.

- Master basic communication skills crucial for patient interviews and history taking.

Topics Covered:

Building Rapport

- **First Impressions:** From the moment the patient walks in, every detail counts, such as greeting them by name and maintaining eye contact. These small gestures contribute to a favourable first impression.

- **Active Listening:** This involves not only hearing what the patient is saying but also understanding it. Use nonverbal cues like nodding to show you're engaged, and avoid interrupting the patient when they're speaking.

- **Empathy and Compassion:** Show genuine concern for the patient's well-being. Empathetic healthcare providers tend to have better patient satisfaction scores and outcomes.

Basic Communication Skills

- **Open-ended Questions:** Start the consultation with open-ended questions like "How can I assist you today?" This allows the patient to express themselves freely and provides the healthcare provider with more comprehensive information.

- **Clarification Techniques:** If a patient provides vague or unclear information, asking for clarification is essential rather than making assumptions. Use follow-up questions or rephrase what you've heard to ensure understanding.

- **Non-verbal Communication:** Pay attention to your body language, which can speak volumes. Maintain an open posture and avoid crossing your arms to appear approachable and receptive.

Case Studies:

Case 1: The Case of Miscommunication

- This case study explores a scenario where poor communication led to an incorrect diagnosis, emphasizing the importance of listening and asking the right questions.

Case 2: Building Rapport in a Sensitive Situation

- A review of a case where a healthcare provider had to deliver difficult news to a patient, focusing on how rapport and effective communication made the situation easier for everyone involved.

Self-Assessment:

- Role-playing exercises for building rapport with different types of patients.

- Multiple-choice questions about effective communication techniques.

Self-Assessment: Enhance Your Communication Skills

1. Role-Playing Exercises for Building Rapport:

Exercise 1: You are a healthcare provider meeting a new patient who is anxious and hesitant. Role-play the initial interaction, focusing on building trust and alleviating the patient's anxiety.

Exercise 2: Imagine you are a healthcare provider dealing with an angry and frustrated patient. Role-play a conversation aimed at de-escalating the situation and addressing the patient's concerns.

Exercise 3: Practice a role-play scenario where you are a healthcare provider interacting with a patient with limited English proficiency. Find effective ways to communicate and ensure the patient's understanding.

2. Multiple-choice questionsBabblingpatients about Effective Communication Techniques:

Question 1: Which of the following is a fundamental component of active listening in healthcare communication?

A) Interrupting the patient to save time.

B) Empathizing with the patient's feelings and concerns.

C) Speaking quickly to ensure all points are covered.

D) Offering unsolicited advice.

Answer: B) Empathizing with the patient's feelings and concerns.

Question 2: True or False: Nonverbal communication, such as maintaining eye contact and using open body language, has no significant impact on the patient-provider relationship.

Answer: False. Nonverbal communication plays a crucial role in building trust and rapport with patients.

Question 3: What is the purpose of using open-ended questions in healthcare communication?

A) To gather specific and concise information from the patient.

B) To guide the conversation toward a predetermined outcome.

C) To encourage the patient to provide detailed information and express their thoughts and feelings.

D) To save time during the patient interview.

Answer: C) To encourage patients to provide detailed information and express their thoughts and feelings.

These self-assessment exercises and questions are designed to help healthcare professionals improve their communication skills, especially in challenging situations. By practicing effective communication techniques, healthcare providers can build better rapport with their patients and provide more patient-centered care.

Summary

Initial patient interaction is not merely a procedural step; it's a critical part of medical practice that can affect everything from diagnosis accuracy to patient satisfaction. Building rapport and employing practical communication skills are beneficial and essential for any healthcare provider committed to offering quality care.

Chapter Six

Identifying Data and Chief Complaints

Introduction

O btaining a medical history begins with gathering essential identifying data and understanding the chief complaint or the primary reason for the patient's visit. This serves as the cornerstone for further diagnostic procedures and treatment plans. This chapter will delve deep into the methodologies and practices for efficiently and effectively gathering this crucial information.

Objectives

- To understand the importance of accurately gathering identifying data.

- To learn techniques for eliciting a precise chief complaint from patients.

- To comprehend how these initial pieces of information can direct the course of diagnosis and treatment.

Topics Covered:

Identifying Data

- **Basic Information:** This includes the patient's name, age, gender, date of birth, address, and contact information. Accurately collecting this data is not just administrative; it's vital for distinguishing between patients and ensuring each individual receives personalized care.

- **Demographics:** Ethnicity, occupation, and marital status can be important for risk assessments and social history. Some conditions are more prevalent in certain demographic groups, and lifestyle factors tied to occupation or marital status may be relevant.

- **Insurance Details:** Necessary for logistical and billing purposes but also crucial for understanding what treatments might be accessible and affordable for the patient.

Chief Complaint

- **Explicit Statements:** Many patients will explicitly state their chief complaint, like "I have a severe headache." It's essential to document these statements verbatim when possible.

- **Vague Descriptions:** Some patients might offer vague or multiple symptoms like, "I'm just not feeling well." In these cases, guided questioning techniques may be used to zero in on the primary issue.

- **Temporal Factors:** Understanding the symptoms' duration, onset, and cyclic nature can offer valuable diagnostic clues. Questions like "How long have you been feeling this way?" or "Do the symptoms come and go?" can be revealing.

- **Aggravating or Alleviating Factors:** Knowing what makes the symptoms worse or better can help narrow potential diagnoses and be critical for immediate treatment options.

Case Studies:

Case 1: The Importance of Detailed Identifying Data

- An exploration of a case where similar names led to a near-miss in diagnosis, emphasizing the crucial role of accurate identifying data.

Case 2: Deciphering a Vague Chief Complaint

- A step-by-step walkthrough of a case where a patient's vague symptoms were carefully dissected through targeted questioning to arrive at a critical diagnosis.

Self-Assessment:

- Multiple-choice quiz on the legal and ethical guidelines surrounding identifying data collection.

- Scenario-based questions on how to handle vague or complicated chief complaints.

Multiple-Choice Quiz on Legal and Ethical Guidelines Surrounding Identifying Data

1. Which of the following documents primarily governs patient privacy and the protection of medical information in the United States?

   ○ A) HIPAA

   ○ B) AMA Code of Ethics

   ○ C) FDA Regulations

   ○ D) Common Law

2. At what point should informed consent be obtained when collecting identifying data?

   ○ A) Before the data is collected

- B) After the data is collected

- C) During the collection of data

- D) Informed consent is not necessary for collecting identifying data

3. Who is allowed to access a patient's identifying data?

  - A) Only the healthcare provider

  - B) Any staff member in the healthcare facility

  - C) Only those who need the information for the care of the patient

  - D) Anyone who asks

4. Failure to adequately protect patient-identifying data could result in the following:

  - A) Legal consequences

  - B) Ethical consequences

  - C) Both legal and ethical consequences

  - D) No consequences

5. What should a healthcare provider do if a patient refuses to provide identifying data?

  - A) Refuse to treat the patient

  - B) Treat the patient but document the refusal

○ C) Seek legal advice before proceeding

○ D) Inform the patient about the risks and implications of not providing the data

Scenario-Based Questions on Handling Vague or Complicated Chief Complaints

1. **Scenario 1**: A patient says, "I'm just not feeling like myself lately." What approach would you take to specify the chief complaint?

2. **Scenario 2**: A patient presents unrelated symptoms like headaches, digestive issues, and fatigue. How would you prioritize and get to the root issue?

3. **Scenario 3**: A patient hesitates to disclose symptoms due to embarrassment. How would you create a comfortable environment for the patient to share openly?

4. **Scenario 4**: A patient cannot provide their chief complaint due to cognitive issues. What are alternative methods for understanding why they sought medical care?

5. **Scenario 5**: A child is brought in by parents who disagree about the main issue. How do you navigate such a situation to determine the actual chief complaint?

These self-assessment tools reinforce your understanding of the legal and ethical aspects of collecting identifying data and handling complex or vague chief complaints. Reviewing your responses will help ensure you are well-equipped to navigate these critical aspects of patient care.

Answers:

Multiple-Choice Quiz on Legal and Ethical Guidelines Surrounding Identifying Data

1. **Answer: A) HIPAA**

   HIPAA (Health Insurance Portability and Accountability Act) is the primary legal framework governing patient privacy and the protection of medical information in the United States.

2. **Answer: A) Before the data is collected**

   Informed consent should be obtained before medical data, including identifying data, is collected to ensure patients understand how their information will be used and protected.

3. **Answer: C) Only those who need the information for the care of the patient**

   Access to identifying data should be restricted to those healthcare providers and staff who require the information to provide proper care.

4. **Answer: C) Both legal and ethical consequences**

   Failure to protect patient data could result in legal repercussions like fines and ethical consequences that may affect licensure or professional standing.

5. **Answer: D) Inform the patient about the risks and implications of not providing the data.**

While collecting identifying data is critical, your feelings are essential entirely; patients have a right to refuse. The healthcare provider should inform the patient about potential risks and document the refusal.

Scenario-Based Questions on Handling Vague or Complicated Chief Complaints

1. **Answer**: For a vague statement like "I'm just not feeling like myself," open-ended questions should be used to encourage the patient to elaborate. You could ask, "Can you tell me more about ?"

2. **Answer**: When a patient presents with multiple symptoms, it's important to prioritize by asking questions like, "Which symptom is causing you the most discomfort?" or "Which symptom appeared first?"

3. **Answer**: To encourage a patient who's embarrassed to disclose symptoms, assure them of confidentiality and that it's a safe space. Explicitly state that their information will not be shared and that understanding fully is essential for proper care.

4. **Answer**: If a patient has cognitive issues and can't articulate their chief complaint, you may need to rely on observations, medical history, and input from family or caregivers.

5. **Answer**: In a case where parents disagree on the child's chief complaint, it may be beneficial to separate them briefly to obtain individual perspectives, and then use medical exper-

tise to decide on the priority for examination.

Summary

Identifying data and the chief complaint in medical practice cannot be overstated. These initial bits of information are not merely routine; they set the trajectory for all subsequent diagnostic and therapeutic steps. Mastery of the techniques for collecting this data efficiently and accurately is essential for any healthcare provider aiming to offer high-quality care.

Chapter Seven

History of Present Illness (HPI)

Introduction

The History of Present Illness (HPI) is a detailed narrative that is the backbone of a patient's medical history. It provides insights into the current complaint and lays the framework for differential diagnosis and treatment plans. This chapter will explore the art and science of effectively collecting the HPI by focusing on detailed questioning and the importance of the chronological order of symptoms.

Objectives

- To understand the fundamental components that make up the HPI.

- To develop skills in conducting detailed interviews for symptom chronology.

- To recognize the value of the HPI in establishing the timeline of a patient's illness, thereby aiding in diagnosis and treatment.

Topics Covered:

Detailed Questioning

- **Open-ended vs. Closed-ended Questions**: Knowing when to use open-ended questions to allow the patient to freely express themselves and when to use closed-ended questions to obtain specific information.

- **The Seven Symptom Attributes** are location, Quality, Quantity or Severity, Timing (including onset, duration, and frequency), Setting, Aggravating/Relief factors, and Associated symptoms (LQQRSTA).

- **Patient's Own Words**: The importance of documenting symptoms as described by the patient, without translating them into medical jargon.

Chronological Order of Symptoms

- **I created a Timeline**: How to guide the patient in describing the order of symptom occurrence, including what led up to it and any fluctuations or progressions.

- **Intersecting Illnesses**: When symptoms might be related to multiple conditions and how to segregate them for a more precise clinical picture.

- **Temporality and Diagnosis**: Understanding the time sequence can offer critical clues in differential diagnosis.

Case Studies:

Case 1: The Case of Evolving Symptoms

- A patient initially presented with mild fatigue and was later discovered to have a complex medical condition. The HPI played a crucial role in connecting the dots.

Case 2: The Misleading Symptom Chronology

- A patient whose symptoms appeared to fit one diagnosis but eventually led to another, underscoring the importance of a meticulous HPI.

Self-Assessment:

- Role-playing exercise: Simulate an HPI collection with a partner.

- Multiple-choice questions to test understanding of the Seven Attributes of a Symptom.

Role-Playing Exercise: Simulate an HPI collection with a partner

In this exercise, one person will act as the healthcare provider, and the other will serve as the patient. The "patient" will have a pre-determined set of symptoms for a hypothetical illness. The "healthcare provider" will conduct the HPI by asking detailed questions to explore the Seven Attributes of a Symptom (LQQRSTA).

Objective:

To practice gathering a detailed and chronological account of a patient's symptoms, paying close attention to open-ended and closed-ended questions.

Scenarios:

- Scenario 1: A patient with abdominal pain

- Scenario 2: A patient with a persistent cough

- Scenario 3: A patient experiencing fatigue and shortness of breath

Switch roles and repeat the exercise for a well-rounded experience.

Multiple-Choice Questions to Test Understanding of the Seven Attributes of a Symptom (LQQRSTA)

1. Which attribute deals with the patient's location of discomfort or pain?

   ○ A) Quality

   ○ B) Location

○ C) Setting

○ D) Timing

2. What does the "Q" in LQQRSTA stand for?

   ○ A) Quantity

   ○ B) Quickness

   ○ C) Quality

   ○ D) Query

3. When asking about "Setting," what are you trying to discover?

   ○ A) The emotional state of the patient

   ○ B) Where was the patient when the symptoms started

   ○ C) The time of day the symptom occurs

   ○ D) How severe the symptom is

4. "Associated symptoms" refers to:

   ○ A) Symptoms that are entirely unrelated but worth noting

   ○ B) Additional symptoms that appear along with the chief complaint

   ○ C) Symptoms that have been ruled out through preliminary tests

○ D) The opposite symptoms of the chief complaint

5. What does the "T" in LQQRSTA stand for?

○ A) Triggering factors

○ B) Temperature

○ C) Timing

○ D) Tolerance

Answers:

1. B) Location

2. C) Quality

3. B) Where was the patient when the symptoms started

4. B) Additional symptoms that appear along with the chief complaint

5. C) Timing

These self-assessment tools should help you reinforce the concepts and skills needed to conduct an effective HPI, which is crucial for accurate diagnosis and treatment planning.

Summary

The History of Present Illness is more than just a recording of symptoms; it is an intricate story that holds clues to diagnosis and treatment. Learning the art of detailed questioning and understanding the chronology of symptoms can be the difference between an accurate diagnosis and a missed one. A well-conducted HPI is thus not just an academic exercise but a critical skill for quality patient care.

Chapter Eight

Past Medical History (PMH)

Introduction

P ast Medical History (PMH) serves as a comprehensive archive of a patient's health status and experiences, offering invaluable insights into diagnosing and managing current health concerns. This chapter will thoroughly understandis collecting and interpreting PMH, including details about previous illnesses, surgeries, hospitalizations, and family history.

Objectives

- Understand the significance of PMH in patient assessment.

- Learn how to obtain information about previous illnesses, surgeries, and hospitalizations.

- Recognize the role of family history in assessing genetic and lifestyle risks.

Topics Covered

Previous Illnesses, Surgeries, and Hospitalizations

- **Chronic Illnesses**: How to inquire about ongoing or recurrent illnesses, their treatment, and any complications.

- **Acute Illnesses**: When and how to discuss past episodes of critical illness, including relevant details such as treatment and recovery time.

- **Surgeries**: Questions to ask about surgical history, such as type of surgery, reason, complications, and post-operative care.

- **Hospitalizations**: Extract critical details about any previous hospital stays, such as length of visit, treatment received, and any complications.

Family History

- **Immediate Family**: The importance of gathering health information about first-degree relatives like parents, siblings, and children.

- **Extended Family**: It's helpful to extend inquiries to aunts, uncles, and grandparents, especially for conditions with known genetic predispositions.

- **Genetic Conditions**: How to probe for hereditary conditions like cancer, diabetes, and cardiovascular disease, among others.

- **Lifestyle Risks**: Learning about familial habits such as diet, exercise, and substance use that could impact the patient's health.

Case Studies:

Case 1: The Impact of PMH in Chronic Disease Management

- How an accurate PMH successfully managed a patient with multiple chronic conditions.

Case 2: The Missing Link in Family History

- This case emphasizes the need for thorough family history-taking, which led to the early detection of a hereditary condition.

Self-Assessment:

- **Fill-in-the-blank questions** about what to include in

PMH.

- **Case scenarios** where you have to identify what parts of the PMH are most relevant to the patient's current condition.

Fill-in-the-Blank Questions:

1. When discussing PMH, it is essential to inquire about _____ illnesses, such as diabetes or hypertension.

2. Information about past _____ is crucial to know if the patient has had any surgical interventions and their outcomes.

3. You must also consider the patient's _____ history, especially the health status of immediate family members like parents, siblings, and children.

4. _____ conditions, such as heart disease or diabetes, that run in the family must be noted in PMH.

5. For a more holistic understanding, one may also consider _____ risks like diet, smoking, and exercise habits in the family.

Case Scenarios:

Scenario 1:

A 45-year-old woman comes into the clinic complaining of abdominal pain. She has no known allergies and is not currently on any medication.

Question:

What parts of her PMH would be most relevant to ask about?

Scenario 2:

A 30-year-old male is concerned about his risk of cardiovascular disease because his father had a heart attack at age 50.

Question:

What aspects of his PMH should you delve into more deeply?

Answers:

Fill-in-the-Blank:

1. Chronic

2. Surgeries

3. Family

4. Genetic

5. Lifestyle

Case Scenarios:

Scenario 1:

In this case, relevant parts of the PMH would include:

- Previous episodes of abdominal pain or gastrointestinal issues

- Any surgeries related to the gastrointestinal system

- Family history of gastrointestinal diseases, if applicable

Scenario 2:

Given the familial history of heart attack, it would be crucial to investigate:

- The patient's history of cardiovascular risk factors like hypertension, diabetes, or high cholesterol

- Family history of cardiovascular disease, including at what age family members were affected

- Lifestyle factors that may contribute to cardiovascular risk, such as diet, exercise, and smoking habits

Through these self-assessment questions and case scenarios, you can evaluate your ability to prioritize and collect essential PMH data for diagnostic and treatment purposes.

Summary

PMH is an integral part of the medical history, providing a holistic view of the patient's health over time. A carefully obtained PMH can offer clues to diagnosing and managing current health issues. This chapter has equipped you with the knowledge and tools to collect and interpret PMH effectively.

Chapter Nine

Review of Systems (ROS)

Introduction

The Review of Systems (ROS) systematically evaluates the patient's overall health by inquiring about different body systems. This is a crucial part of the patient assessment and should not be hurried. By asking comprehensive questions about each body system, clinicians can better understand a patient's health status.

Objectives

- Understand the significance of the ROS in patient diagnosis and management.

- Learn how to inquire about various body systems systematically.

- Recognize which details are pertinent in specific scenarios.

Topics Covered

Comprehensive Questioning about Body Systems

- **General System**: Weight loss, fatigue, fever.

- **Skin and Hair**: Rashes, itching, changes in hair or nails.

- **Head and Neck**: Headaches, vision issues, neck stiffness.

- **Cardiovascular**: Chest pain, shortness of breath, edema.

- **Respiratory**: Cough, wheezing, sputum production.

- **Gastrointestinal**: Nausea, vomiting, diarrhea, constipation.

- **Genitourinary**: Frequency, urgency, dysuria.

- **Musculoskeletal**: Muscle or joint pain, stiffness, swelling.

- **Neurological**: Tremors, seizures, numbness.

- **Psychiatric**: Anxiety, depression, hallucinations.

- **Endocrine**: Heat or cold intolerance, polyuria, polydipsia.

- **Hematologic**: Easy bruising, history of anemia or clotting disorders.

Case Studies:

Case 1: The Importance of ROS in Complex Cases

- How a meticulous ROS revealed underlying cardiovascular and gastrointestinal issues in a patient with multiple complaints.

Case 2: The Pitfall of Skipping ROS

- A case demonstrating the adverse consequences of skipping or rushing the ROS, leading to a misdiagnosis.

Self-Assessment:

- **Multiple-choice questions** on how to structure the ROS for different patient profiles.

- **Role-playing exercise**: Practicing the ROS questioning with a partner.

Self-Assessment:

Multiple-Choice Questions:

1. When a patient complains of general fatigue and weight loss, which systems should be given particular attention in the ROS?

    ○ A) Gastrointestinal and Endocrine

    ○ B) Cardiovascular and Respiratory

    ○ C) Musculoskeletal and Neurological

    ○ D) Skin and Hair

2. A young adult reports frequent headaches. Which additional body systems should be closely reviewed in the ROS?

    ○ A) Cardiovascular and Respiratory

    ○ B) Neurological and Psychiatric

    ○ C) Gastrointestinal and Genitourinary

    ○ D) Hematologic and Musculoskeletal

3. An elderly patient with a history of heart disease comes in for a routine check-up. Which systems are crucial to include in the ROS?

    ○ A) Cardiovascular and Respiratory

    ○ B) General and Endocrine

    ○ C) Skin and Hair

    ○ D) Genitourinary and Neurological

4. A patient reports joint pain and stiffness. Which other body

systems should be evaluated in the ROS?

- ○ A) Respiratory and Cardiovascular

- ○ B) Musculoskeletal and Neurological

- ○ C) Gastrointestinal and Genitourinary

- ○ D) Hematologic and Endocrine

Role-Playing Exercise:

Scenario 1:
You are the healthcare provider, and your partner is a patient who has come in complaining of frequent stomach upset and changes in bowel habits.

- • Practice asking comprehensive ROS questions that include inquiries into the Gastrointestinal, Endocrine, and General systems. Note any relevant findings.

Scenario 2:
Now, swap roles. Your partner is the healthcare provider; you are a patient who has come in for an annual check-up with no specific complaints.

- • Your partner should practice conducting a comprehensive ROS covering multiple body systems.

Answers:

Multiple-Choice Questions:

1. A) Gastrointestinal and Endocrine: These systems are often related to symptoms like fatigue and weight loss.

2. B) Neurological and Psychiatric: Headaches can be related to neurological issues, stress, and anxiety.

3. A) Cardiovascular and Respiratory: Given the patient's history of heart disease, these systems should be reviewed closely.

4. B) Musculoskeletal and Neurological: Joint pain can be linked to musculoskeletal issues and neurological conditions like neuropathy.

By completing this self-assessment, you can effectively validate your understanding of how to customize the Review of Systems according to varying patient profiles.

Summary

The Review of Systems (ROS) is an indispensable tool for healthcare providers. By examining the patient through the lens of multiple body systems, the ROS offers a layered, comprehensive view of the patient's health. As a healthcare provider, understanding how to conduct the ROS properly can significantly aid in the accuracy of your diagnosis and subsequent care management.

Chapter Ten

The General Survey

Introduction

The General Survey is the initial phase of the physical examination and serves as an essential guidepost for the more detailed evaluations that follow. It encompasses the vital signs and an assessment of the patient's overall appearance, including aspects like hygiene, cognitive state, and distress levels. This first impression often provides vital clues about the patient's overall health status.

Objectives

- Recognize the importance of conducting a comprehensive General Survey.

- Understand how to accurately measure vital signs.

- Assess the patient's overall appearance for significant indicators of health or illness.

Topics Covered

Vital Signs

- **Temperature**: Methods of measurement and normal ranges

- **Blood Pressure**: Procedure for accurate measurement and interpretation of readings

- **Heart Rate**: How to count and what to look for in rhythm and regularity

- **Respiratory Rate**: Counting and significance of different rates

- **Oxygen Saturation**: Importance and how to measure

Overall Appearance

- **Hygiene**: Assessment of cleanliness and grooming

- **Nutritional Status**: Signs of malnutrition or obesity

- **Facial Expression**: Observing for signs of distress, pain, or anxiety

- **Posture and Gait**: Evaluation of body mechanics

- **Skin Color and Texture**: Checking for signs of pallor, cyanosis, or jaundice

Temperature: Methods of Measurement and Normal Ranges

Methods of Measurement

- **Oral**: Measured under the tongue; most common for adults.

- **Axillary**: Measured under the armpit; often used for children.

- **Tympanic**: Measured in the ear; quick but less accurate.

- **Rectal**: Measured in the rectum; considered the most accurate.

Normal Ranges

- Adults: 97°F (36.1°C) to 99°F (37.2°C)

- Children: 97.8°F (36.5°C) to 98.6°F (37°C)

Blood Pressure: Procedure for Accurate Measurement and Interpretation of Readings

Procedure

1. Seat the patient and ensure they are relaxed for at least 5 minutes.

2. Use an appropriately sizedBody Mechanicsto measure vital signs accuratelyhealthcriticalsized bod cuff; too small can give falsely high readings.

3. Place the cuff on the bare upper arm.

4. Measure at heart level.

5. Inflate the cuff while listening with a stethoscope.

6. Note the systolic and diastolic pressures.

Interpretation

- Normal: Below 120/80 mm Hg

- Elevated: 120-129/<80 mm Hg

- Hypertension Stage 1: 130-139/80-89 mm Hg

- Hypertension Stage 2: 140+/90+ mm Hg

Heart Rate: How to Count and What to Look for in Rhythm and Regularity

Counting

- Use a stopwatch or second hand and count beats for 15 seconds, then multiply by 4.

Rhythm and Regularity

- A regular rhythm has consistent beats.

- An irregular rhythm has inconsistent beats and should be evaluated for arrhythmias.

Respiratory Rate: Counting and Significance of Different Rates

Counting

- Count for one full minute or count for 30 seconds and multiply by 2.

Significance

- Regular: 12-20 breaths per minute

- Tachypnea: Above 20 breaths per minute

- Bradypnea: Below 12 breaths per minute

Oxygen Saturation: Importance and How to Measure

Importance

- Indicates how well oxygen is being delivered to the peripheral tissues.

Measurement

- Use a pulse oximeter placed on a fingertip or earlobe.

Overall Appearance

Hygiene

- Look for signs of grooming and cleanliness, as poor hygiene may signify neglect or psychiatric issues.

Nutritional Status

- Assess weight, body mass index, and any signs of malnutrition or obesity.

Facial Expression

- Observe for grimacing, tension, or other signs of distress, pain, or anxiety.

Posture and Gait

- Look for abnormal curvature, limping, or other irregularities that could signal underlying issues.

Skin Color and Texture

- Check for pallor (pale), cyanosis (blue), or jaundice (yellow), which can be indicators of systemic conditions.

Considering all these elements during a physical exam, you'll gather invaluable information to guide diagnosis and treatment.

Case Studies:

Case 1: The Misleading Vital Signs

- A story highlighted the importance of considering vital signs and overall appearance, where normal vitals masked a more severe underlying condition.

Case 2: The Telltale Signs of Distress

- A case where the patient's overall appearance revealed significant distress, prompting a more thorough investigation.

Case 1: The Misleading Vital Signs

Scenario

Nurse Sarah was evaluating a 45-year-old man who came to the emergency room with complaints of generalized fatigue. The vital signs were as follows:

- Temperature: 98.6°F

- Blood Pressure: 120/80 mm Hg

- Heart Rate: 75 bpm

- Respiratory Rate: 18 breaths/min

- Oxygen Saturation: 98%

At a glance, the vital signs looked perfectly normal, fitting comfortably within the standard ranges. However, Nurse Sarah noticed the patient had a pallor complexion and appeared lethargic. Upon a closer look, she also found the mask accurately. It is a hypocritical-sized body mechanism that his nails had a blue tinge.

Action and Outcome

Trusting her instincts and the importance of considering overall appearance alongside vitals, Sarah ordered an immediate blood test. The results revealed severe anemia, contributing to the patient's symptoms and explained the bluish nails, a sign of hypoxia. Immediate treatment was initiated, and the patient was hospitalized for further evaluation and management.

Lesson

This case highlights the importance of looking beyond just the numbers. Vital signs may sometimes appear normal, even when a patient is experiencing a significant medical issue. Always consider the overall appearance and other subtle cues.

Case 2: The Telltale Signs of Distress

Scenario

Dr. Williams was doing rounds in the general ward when he encountered a 30-year-old woman admitted for abdominal pain. Her vital signs were slightly elevated but not alarmingly so:

- Temperature: 99°F

- Blood Pressure: 128/85 mm Hg

- Heart Rate: 90 bpm

- Respiratory Rate: 22 breaths/min

- Oxygen Saturation: 97%

However, her face was contorted in pain, she appeared anxious, and her posture was rigid, indicating distress.

Action and Outcome

Despite the borderline ordinary vital signs, Dr. Williams was prompted by her appearance to dig deeper. Additional diagnostic tests, including an abdominal ultrasound, were ordered immediately. The ultrasound revealed gallstones, leading to a diagnosis of acute cholecystitis. The patient underwent surgery shortly after and recovered well.

Lesson

The patient's overall appearance and body language were crucial in revealing the severity of her condition. While the vital signs offered some clues, they did not fully expose her distress. Therefore, always consider subjective factors and the patient's overall demeanour for a more holistic evaluation.

Both cases emphasize the need for a comprehensive approach when evaluating patients, blending clinical measurements and a keen eye for subjective signs of distress or disease.

Self-Assessment:

- **Multiple-choice quiz** on interpreting different sets of vital signs.

- **Role-playing exercise**: Practicing the General Survey with a partner.

Multiple-Choice Quiz:

1. What is considered an average adult resting heart rate?

- ○ A) 40-60 bpm

- ○ B) 60-100 bpm

- ○ C) 100-120 bpm

- ○ D) 120-140 bpm

2. A patient has a blood pressure reading of 135/95 mm Hg. How would you classify this?

- ○ A) Normal

- ○ B) Elevated

- ○ C) Hypertension Stage 1

- ○ D) Hypertension Stage 2

3. What oxygen saturation level generally requires immediate intervention?

- ○ A) Above 98%

- ○ B) 94-98%

- ○ C) 90-93%

- ○ D) Below 90%

4. A respiratory rate of 22 breaths per minute in a resting adult is:

- ○ A) Normal

- ○ B) Bradypnea

- ○ C) Tachypnea

- ○ D) Hyperpnea

Role-Playing Exercise:

Scenario 1:

You are the healthcare provider, and your partner is a patient who has come in for a routine check-up.

- Practice taking your partner's "vital signs," such as blood pressure, heart rate, and respiratory rate. Also, observe their overall appearance and hygiene. Discuss your findings.

Scenario 2:

Switch roles. Now, your partner is the healthcare provider, and you are the patient who has come in due to general fatigue and occasional dizzy spells.

- Your partner should practice conducting a General Survey, taking into account your "symptoms" to perform a more targeted assessment.

Answers:

Multiple-Choice Quiz:

1. B) 60-100 bpm: This is adults' average resting heart rateconsiderin.

2. C) Hypertension Stage 1: A blood pressure reading of 135/95 mm Hg is considered in the range of Hypertension Stage 1.

3. D) Below 90%: Oxygen saturation levels below 90% typically require immediate intervention.

4. C) Tachypnea: A respiratory rate of 22 breaths per minute in a resting adult is considered tachypneic.

Completing this self-assessment will enhance your understanding of conducting and interpreting a comprehensive General Survey, which is crucial in clinical practice.

Summary

The General Survey is a fundamental part of the physical examination process. Accurately taking vital signs and making astute observations about the patient's overall appearance can direct the healthcare provider toward a more accurate diagnosis and effective treatment plan. It is a skill that improves with practice and attentiveness to detail.

Chapter Eleven

Head and Neck Examination

Introduction

T he head and neck examination is a critical component of a comprehensive physical assessment, offering clues into a variety of systemic and localized issues. From eyesight and hearing to potential neurological or endocrine issues, this section of the exam can be incredibly revealing.

Objectives

- Understand the significance of a thorough head and neck examination.

- Master the techniques involved in examining the eyes, ears, nose, and throat.

- Recognize common abnormalities and their implications.

Topics Covered

Examination of Eyes

Importance: Eyes are the windows to a variety of systemic diseases such as diabetes, hypertension, and even neurologic disorders.

Techniques:

- **Visual Acuity**: Testing clarity of vision using a Snellen chart.

- **Ophthalmoscopic Examination**: Using an ophthalmoscope to inspect the interior surface of the eye.

- **Conjunctival and Scleral Assessment**: Checking for pallor or jaundice.

- **Pupil Examination**: Inspecting size, shape, and reactivity to light.

Common Abnormalities: Cataracts, glaucoma, retinal detachment.

Examination of Ears

Importance: Ears are not just auditory organs; issues here could relate to balance or even systemic infections.

Techniques:

- **Inspect External Ear**: Look for deformities, lumps, or signs of infection.

- **Otoscope Examination**: Use an otoscope to examine the

ear canal and tympanic membrane.

- **Audiometry**: Testing hearing acuity.

Common Abnormalities: Otitis media, hearing loss, tinnitus.

Examination of Nose

Importance: The nose is an entry point for respiratory systems; issues here could indicate allergies, infections, or other respiratory issues.

Techniques:

- **External Inspection**: Observe for symmetry and deformities.

- **Internal Examination**: Using a light source to inspect the nasal passages.

Common Abnormalities: Deviated septum, nasal polyps, signs of rhinitis.

Examination of Throat

Importance: Throat issues can be signs of systemic infection, allergic reactions, or gastrointestinal issues.

Techniques:

- **Inspect Oral Cavity**: Using a tongue depressor and light, inspect the gums, teeth, tongue, and palate.

- **Tonsil Examination**: Check for enlargement, redness, or signs of infection.

- **Gag Reflex**: Testing the integrity of cranial nerves.

Common Abnormalities: Tonsillitis, oral thrush, signs of gastroesophageal reflux disease (GERD).

Self-Assessment

- **Multiple-choice quiz on recognizing eye abnormalities through descriptions.**

- **Scenario-based questions on what to do if you encounter specific ear abnormalities.**

Multiple-Choice Quiz on Recognizing Eye Abnormalities Through Descriptions

1. **Which of the following might indicate glaucoma?**

   ○ A. A "halo" effect around lights

   ○ B. Double vision

   ○ C. Yellowing of the sclera

   ○ D. Night blindness

2. **A patient complains of "floaters" and flashing lights in their vision. What could this be a symptom of?**

   ○ A. Retinal detachment

   ○ B. Cataract

   ○ C. Astigmatism

○ D. Hyperopia

3. **What does a pale optic disc during an ophthalmoscopic examination usually indicate?**

○ A. Optic neuritis

○ B. Healthy optic nerve

○ C. Glaucoma

○ D. Macular degeneration

Scenario-Based Questions on What to Do if You Encounter Specific Ear Abnormalities

1. **You notice an inflamed and red tympanic membrane during an otoscope examination. What is the likely diagnosis and what should be your next step?**

Likely Diagnosis
: Acute otitis media
Next Step
: Confirm the diagnosis with further tests if needed, and discuss antibiotic treatment options with the physician.

2. **The patient complains of a constant buzzing sound in the ears but shows no signs of infection or blockage. What could this be indicative of, and what should you do?**

Likely Diagnosis
: Tinnitus

Next Step

: Refer the patient for a full audiological evaluation and consult the physician for potential underlying causes such as hypertension or medications.

3. **You see a yellowish discharge coming from a patient's ear. What is the likely diagnosis and what should be the next course of action?**

Likely Diagnosis

: Otitis externa (Swimmer's Ear)

Next Step

: Clean the ear carefully, take a sample for culture if necessary, and consult the physician for antibiotic ear drops.

By completing this self-assessment, you'll be better equipped to identify common abnormalities during a head and neck examination and will know how to proceed effectively.

Summary

The head and neck examination is a comprehensive and vital component of overall patient evaluation. A variety of systemic issues may first become evident here, making this examination a critical part of medical practice.

Chapter Twelve

Respiratory Examination

Introduction

The respiratory examination is a critical element of the total patient assessment, crucial for diagnosing conditions ranging from common respiratory infections to more severe issues like pleural effusion or lung cancer. This chapter provides a comprehensive guide to conducting a respiratory examination effectively.

Objectives

- Understand the significance of a thorough respiratory examination.

- Master the techniques involved in lung auscultation, inspection, and palpation.

- Recognize common respiratory abnormalities and their implications.

Topics Covered

Lung Auscultation

Importance: Auscultation can reveal much about lung function and is crucial for diagnosing pneumonia, asthma, and COPD.

Techniques:

- **Normal Breath Sounds**: Understanding vesicular, bronchial, and tracheal breath sounds.

- **Adventitious Sounds**: Recognizing wheezes, crackles, and pleural rubs.

- **Equipment**: Proper use of a stethoscope, including diaphragm and bell.

Common Abnormalities: Wheezing in asthma, crackles in pneumonia, absent breath sounds in pneumothorax.

Inspection of the Respiratory System

Importance: Visual cues often offer the first signs of respiratory issues, such as rapid rate, use of accessory muscles, or cyanosis.

Techniques:

- **Chest Symmetry**: Looking for deformities or asymmetry in chest expansion.

- **Skin and Lip Color**: Checking for pallor or cyanosis.

- **Respiratory Rate and Pattern**: Noting any irregularities.

Common Abnormalities: Barrel chest in COPD, cyanosis in hypoxia, rapid breathing in respiratory distress.

Palpation of the Chest

Importance: Palpation can help assess chest expansion, tenderness, and tactile fremitus.

Techniques:

- **Chest Expansion**: Hands-on assessment to gauge symmetry of chest movement.

- **Tactile Fremitus**: Using hands to feel for vibrations during speech.

Common Abnormalities: Decreased expansion in pleural effusion, increased fremitus in pneumonia.

Self-Assessment

- **Multiple-choice quiz on distinguishing between different adventitious lung sounds.**

- **Scenario-based questions on how to interpret findings from chest palpation.**

Multiple-Choice Quiz on Distinguishing Between Different Adventitious Lung Sounds

1. **Which lung sound is commonly heard in asthma patients?**

   ◦ A. Crackles

   ◦ B. Wheezing

   ◦ C. Stridor

   ◦ D. Pleural Rub

2. **What adventitious sound is commonly associated with pneumonia?**

   ◦ A. Rhonchi

   ◦ B. Crackles

   ◦ C. Wheezing

   ◦ D. Tracheal sounds

3. **Which lung sound might you expect in a patient with a large pleural effusion?**

   ◦ A. Increased vesicular sounds

   ◦ B. Absent breath sounds

   ◦ C. Rhonchi

   ◦ D. Wheezing

Scenario-Based Questions on How to Interpret Findings From Chest Palpation

1. **You palpate a patient's chest who complains of localized pain on the right side. You notice that tactile fremitus is increased on that side. What could this potentially indicate?**

Potential Indication

: This could suggest consolidation of lung tissue, such as might occur with pneumonia or lung mass.

Next Steps

: Further diagnostic tests like X-rays or CT scans should be conducted for a confirmed diagnosis.

2. **During chest palpation, chest expansion is significantly decreased on the left side. What could be the underlying issue?**

Potential Indication

: Decreased chest expansion on one side may indicate pleural effusion, pneumothorax, or a mass compressing the lung.

Next Steps

: Immediate imaging studies are necessary to identify the underlying cause.

3. **You notice crepitus during palpation around the upper chest and neck area. What does this finding usually signify?**

Potential Indication

: Crepitus usually suggests subcutaneous emphysema, often seen in conditions involving air leaks into the subcutaneous tissue, like chest trauma or severe lung infection.

Next Steps

: Immediate medical intervention and imaging studies are essential for diagnosis and treatment planning.

By completing this self-assessment, you'll deepen your understanding of how to conduct a thorough respiratory examination and interpret the findings effectively.

Summary

The respiratory examination is a cornerstone of thorough patient assessment. By mastering these techniques, healthcare professionals can detect various conditions, facilitating early and effective treatment. This chapter is a comprehensive guide for clinicians at all levels, aiming to improve patient outcomes through competent examination practices.

Chapter Thirteen

Cardiovascular Examination

Introduction

The cardiovascular examination is a pivotal component of the overall clinical evaluation, allowing healthcare providers to detect various conditions, from hypertension and arrhythmias to more severe issues like heart failure or valvular heart disease. This chapter will offer a comprehensive guide on conducting an adequate cardiovascular examination.

Objectives

- To understand the critical elements of a cardiovascular examination.

- To learn how to evaluate heart rate, blood pressure, and peripheral circulation.

- To recognize common cardiovascular abnormalities and their clinical significance.

Topics Covered

Heart Rate Assessment

Importance: A fundamental measure of cardiovascular health, variations in heart rate can indicate conditions such as bradycardia or tachycardia.

Techniques:

- **Pulse palpation**: Commonly at the radial or carotid artery.

- **Use of a stethoscope**: For auscultation of the heart to assess rhythm and regularity.

Common Abnormalities: Arrhythmias like atrial fibrillation and ventricular tachycardia.

Blood Pressure Measurement

Importance: Blood pressure is a critical cardiovascular risk and organ perfusion indicator.

Techniques:

- **Selection of appropriate cuff size**: To ensure accurate measurement.

- **Correct positioning**: Arm at heart level, both feet on the ground.

- **Sequential measurements**: To account for white-coat syndrome or other transient factors.

Common Abnormalities: Hypertension, hypotension, orthostatic changes.

Peripheral Circulation

Importance: Assessment of peripheral circulation can offer clues about systemic circulatory issues or localized vascular problems.

Techniques:

- **Capillary refill time**: A quick test for peripheral perfusion.

- **Pulse examination**: In various locations to assess for pulse symmetry and strength.

Common Abnormalities: Peripheral arterial disease, deep vein thrombosis.

Self-Assessment

- **Multiple-choice quiz on common conditions that can alter heart rate.**

- **Scenario-based questions on how to interpret abnormal blood pressure readings.**

Multiple-Choice Quiz on Common Conditions That Can Alter Heart Rate

1. **Which condition is most likely to result in tachycardia?**

    ◦ A. Hypothyroidism

    ◦ B. Hyperthyroidism

    ◦ C. Hypothermia

    ◦ D. Sedative overdose

2. **Bradycardia is most commonly associated with:**

    ◦ A. Anxiety

    ◦ B. Beta-blocker medications

    ◦ C. Fever

    ◦ D. Dehydration

3. **Which electrolyte imbalance can lead to arrhythmias?**

    ◦ A. Hypercalcemia

    ◦ B. Hypokalemia

    ◦ C. Hypernatremia

    ◦ D. Hypermagnesemia

Scenario-Based Questions on How to Interpret Abnormal Blood Pressure Readings

1. You measure a patient's blood pressure and find 180/110 mm Hg. The patient is asymptomatic. What is your next course of action?

Potential Interpretation

: This could be a hypertensive crisis, even if the patient is asymptomatic.

Next Steps

: Immediate re-measurement, followed by appropriate medical intervention and possibly hospital admission for close monitoring.

2. **A patient presents with a blood pressure of 90/60 mm Hg and reports dizziness upon standing. What could this indicate?**

Potential Interpretation

: This could be orthostatic hypotension.

Next Steps

: Re-measure blood pressure in different positions (sitting, standing, lying down) and consider further evaluation for underlying causes.

3. **Blood pressure is 160/100 mm Hg in a patient with no previous history of hypertension. What is your next step?**

Potential Interpretation

: This could be stage 2 hypertension.

Next Steps

: Confirm with repeated measurements and initiate appropriate diagnostic tests and treatments, possibly including antihypertensive medication.

Completing this self-assessment will allow you to gauge your understanding of the cardiovascular examination and offer practical applications for abnormal findings.

Summary

The cardiovascular examination is a cornerstone in patient assessment for cardiovascular health. Mastering these techniques will provide clinicians at all levels with valuable insights into patient health, facilitating timely diagnosis and effective treatment. This chapter aims to be a comprehensive resource for honing these crucial skills.

Chapter Fourteen

Gastrointestinal Examination

Introduction

The gastrointestinal examination is fundamental to a comprehensive clinical assessment, offering valuable insights into the digestive system and other related organs. This chapter will guide healthcare providers through the techniques and importance of a detailed gastrointestinal examination.

Objectives

- To understand the critical elements of a gastrointestinal examination.

- To learn the techniques for abdominal inspection, auscultation, and palpation.

- To recognize common gastrointestinal abnormalities.

Topics Covered

Abdominal Inspection

Importance: Provides initial clues to conditions such as distension, scarring, or skin changes.

Techniques:

- **Visual Inspection**: Check for symmetry, contour, and any visible masses or scars.

- **Skin Changes**: Note any discoloration, veins, or striae.

Common Abnormalities: Ascites, surgical scars, jaundice.

Abdominal Auscultation

Importance: Evaluating bowel sounds can indicate the function of the gastrointestinal system.

Techniques:

- **Use of Stethoscope**: Listen in all four quadrants of the abdomen for bowel sounds.

- **Frequency and Character**: Note the frequency and character (e.g., gurgling, tinkling, silence).

Common Abnormalities: Hyperactive sounds in gastroenteritis, diminished or absent sounds in ileus or peritonitis.

Abdominal Palpation

Importance: Helps in identifying masses, tenderness, or organ enlargement.

Techniques:

- **Light Palpation**: To assess surface characteristics and tenderness.

- **Deep Palpation**: To feel for deeper structures and masses.

Common Abnormalities: Hepatomegaly, tenderness in acute appendicitis, abdominal masses.

Self-Assessment

- **Multiple-choice quiz on common reasons for abdominal distension.**

- **Scenario-based questions on how to interpret various types of bowel sounds.**

Multiple-Choice Quiz on Common Reasons for Abdominal Distension

1. **Which of the following is a common cause of acute abdominal distension?**

   - A. Irritable Bowel Syndrome (IBS)

   - B. Ascites

- ○ C. Gastric outlet obstruction

- ○ D. Constipation

2. **Chronic abdominal distension is most often related to:**

- ○ A. Acute pancreatitis

- ○ B. Irritable Bowel Syndrome (IBS)

- ○ C. Peritonitis

- ○ D. Acute appendicitis

3. **In which condition is abdominal distension commonly associated with jaundice?**

- ○ A. Cholecystitis

- ○ B. Hepatic cirrhosis

- ○ C. Acute gastritis

- ○ D. Small bowel obstruction

Scenario-Based Questions on How to Interpret Various Types of Bowel Sounds

1. **You hear high-pitched tinkling sounds during abdominal auscultation. What might you suspect?**

Potential Interpretation
: This type of sound is commonly associated with bowel obstruction.

Next Steps

: Consider further diagnostic imaging such as an abdominal X-ray or CT scan and consult with a surgical team for potential intervention.

2. **You auscultate the abdomen and hear no bowel sounds for more than 5 minutes. What is your next course of action?**

Potential Interpretation

: Absence of bowel sounds could indicate paralytic ileus or peritonitis.

Next Steps

: Immediate further evaluation is required, including additional imaging and potentially urgent surgical consultation.

3. **During auscultation, you notice the bowel sounds are louder and more frequent than usual. What could this signify?**

Potential Interpretation

: Hyperactive bowel sounds may indicate a condition such as gastroenteritis.

Next Steps

: Consider other symptoms such as diarrhea or vomiting and initiate appropriate treatment, which may include rehydration and anti-emetics.

This self-assessment should help you evaluate your understanding of abdominal distension and interpreting various bowel sounds, thereby improving your ability to make more accurate diagnoses.

Summary

A detailed gastrointestinal examination is indispensable for diagnosing various disorders related to digestion, excretion, and other organ systems like the cardiovascular and endocrine systems. This chapter aims to serve as a comprehensive guide for conducting these evaluations effectively.

Chapter Fifteen

Neurological Examination

Introduction

The neurological examination is a critical component of the general physical examination and is essential in assessing the integrity of a patient's central and peripheral nervous systems. This chapter aims to guide healthcare providers in performing a thorough neurological evaluation, focusing on reflexes, coordination, and sensory function.

Objectives

- To understand the critical components of a neurological examination.

- To learn how to assess reflexes, coordination, and sensory function effectively.

- To recognize common neurological disorders.

Topics Covered

Reflexes

Importance: Reflexes serve as an initial indicator of the integrity of the nervous system.

Techniques:

- **Deep Tendon Reflexes**: Use a reflex hammer to test reflexes like the patellar reflex (knee-jerk) or the Achilles reflex.

- **Superficial Reflexes**: Assess reflexes like the abdominal reflex and the corneal reflex.

Common Abnormalities: Hyperreflexia, hyporeflexia, areflexia.

Coordination

Importance: Tests the cerebellar function and upper motor neuron integrity.

Techniques:

- **Finger-to-Nose Test**: The patient uses the tip of the index finger to touch the nose.

- **Heel-Shin Test**: The patient is asked to slide the heel of one foot along the shin of the other leg.

Common Abnormalities: Ataxia, tremors, dysmetria.

Sensory Function

Importance: Evaluates the somatic and visceral senses, contributing to diagnosing peripheral neuropathies and central nervous system disorders.

    Techniques:

- **Pain and Temperature**: Use sharp and dull objects or hot and cold elements to test.

- **Proprioception**: Assess sense of body position.

- **Delicate Touch**: Use a cotton wisp to assess.

    Common Abnormalities: Hypoesthesia, hyperesthesia, allodynia.

Self-Assessment

- **Multiple-choice quiz on the significance of absent or diminished reflexes.**

- **Scenario-based questions on how to interpret coordination test results.**

Multiple-Choice Quiz: Significance of Absent or Diminished Reflexes

1. What does hyporeflexia generally indicate?

a) An overactive nervous system

b) No particular significance

c) Possible peripheral nerve damage

d) Upper motor neuron disorder

   2. An absent Achilles reflex may be indicative of:

a) Cerebellar damage

b) S1-S2 nerve root dysfunction

c) Hypothyroidism

d) Hyperactive sympathetic nervous system

   3. A diminished corneal reflex might indicate:

a) Trigeminal nerve dysfunction

b) Hyperactivity of the nervous system

c) Emotional distress

d) Cerebral palsy

Scenario-Based Questions: How to Interpret Coordination Test Results

1. Scenario: A patient exhibits a significant tremor during the Finger-to-Nose test. What could this possibly indicate?

Answer
: A significant tremor during the Finger-to-Nose test might be indicative of a cerebellar dysfunction or a Parkinsonian syndrome. Immediate further assessment is required.

2. Scenario: During the Heel-Shin test, a patient slides the heel smoothly along the shin without any issues. However, they report discomfort while doing so. How should you interpret these findings?

Answer

: If the patient can perform the Heel-Shin test accurately but reports discomfort, it may indicate a sensory issue rather than a problem with coordination. Additional sensory testing is advised.

    3. Scenario: A patient struggles to maintain balance during any coordination tests, swaying significantly while standing still. What should be your next step in evaluation?

Answer

: Struggling to maintain balance during coordination tests could suggest a vestibular or proprioceptive dysfunction. Referral to a neurologist for comprehensive evaluation is recommended.

Remember, these are just tools to aid your understanding and should not replace a professional evaluation. Always consult with medical professionals for accurate diagnosis and appropriate management.

Summary

A comprehensive neurological examination can provide invaluable insights into a patient's overall health, specifically into their nervous system's integrity. Learning to perform this exam accurately and interpret its results can significantly aid in diagnosing and treating various neurological conditions.

Chapter Sixteen

Musculoskeletal Examination

Topics Covered:

1. **Introduction to Musculoskeletal Examination**: Understanding the importance of assessing joint function, muscle strength, and range of motion.

2. **Preparation**: Necessary patient positioning and examiner's hand techniques for a comprehensive evaluation.

3. **Joint Function**: Techniques for examining joints including:

   - Inspection for deformity, swelling, or color changes

   - Palpation for tenderness or warmth

   - Range of motion tests

   - Stability tests

4. **Muscle Strength**: Understanding the grading scale for muscle strength (0-5) and how to apply it during examination.

5. **Range of Motion (ROM)**: Types of ROM (active, passive, and resistive) and their significance.

   ○ Measuring ROM using a goniometer

   ○ Identifying limitations and comparing them to established norms

6. **Special Tests**: Performing specific musculoskeletal tests like:

   ○ Anterior drawer test for knee stability

   ○ Phalen's test for carpal tunnel syndrome

   ○ Straight leg raise for lumbar radiculopathy

Self-Assessment

Multiple-Choice Quiz: Joint Function and Muscle Strength

1. What does a muscle strength grade of 2 signify?

a) No contraction
b) Full ROM against gravity
c) Full ROM with gravity eliminated
d) Partial ROM against gravity

2. In which condition is the Anterior Drawer Test commonly used?

a) Hip dislocation

b) Ankle sprain

c) Knee injury

d) Elbow fracture

3. Limited ROM in the shoulder could be indicative of:

a) Sciatica

b) Rotator cuff tear

c) Carpal tunnel syndrome

d) Achilles tendon rupture

Scenario-Based Questions: Interpretation of Range of Motion

1. Scenario: A patient cannot flex the elbow beyond 90 degrees. What could this potentially signify?

Answer

: Limited elbow flexion could indicate possible joint pathology like osteoarthritis, or muscle issues such as a bicep strain. Further diagnostic tests may be necessary.

2. Scenario: During the examination, you observe that the patient is unable to perform dorsiflexion of the ankle. What would be your next course of action?

Answer

: Inability to dorsiflex the ankle could be due to a range of issues, from muscle weakness to neurological disorders. Additional testing, possibly including imaging and nerve conduction studies, would be advisable.

3. Scenario: A patient reports difficulty in abducting the arm beyond shoulder height. What might be the underlying issue?

Answer

: Difficulty in arm abduction could indicate a rotator cuff injury, adhesive capsulitis (frozen shoulder), or other shoulder pathologies. Immediate further assessment is required.

Remember, these assessments are just educational tools and should not replace a thorough medical evaluation. Always consult with a healthcare professional for an accurate diagnosis and treatment plan.

Chapter Seventeen

Dermatological Examination

Topics Covered:

1. **Introduction to Dermatological Examination**: Explaining the role of skin assessment in general health and the diagnosis of skin conditions.

2. **Preparation**: Required lighting, patient positioning, and examiner's techniques for a practical dermatological evaluation.

3. **Assessing Skin Appearance**:

   - Colour: Looking for pallor, cyanosis, or jaundice

   - Texture: Assessing for dryness, scaliness, or smoothness

   - Moisture: Noting excessive dryness or moisture

4. Examination of Lesions:

- Type: Identifying if it's a macule, papule, nodule, etc.

- Size: Measuring the dimensions

- Shape: Describing as round, irregular, etc.

- Color: Noting if it's pigmented, erythematous, etc.

- Distribution: Assessing the pattern and location of the body

5. Special Examinations:

- Wood's lamp examination for fungal or bacterial infections

- Tzanck smear for suspected viral lesions like herpes

6. **Dermoscopy:** Using a dermatoscope for more detailed examination of skin lesions.

Self-Assessment

Multiple-Choice Quiz: Understanding Skin Appearance and Lesions

1. What does cyanosis usually indicate?

a) High oxygen levels
b) Low oxygen levels

c) Jaundice

d) Normal skin colour

2. Which of the following lesions is flat and measures less than 1 cm in diameter?

a) Macule

b) Papule

c) Plaque

d) Nodule

3. A patient with a ring-like rash on the arm is most likely suffering from:

a) Psoriasis

b) Ringworm

c) Eczema

d) Vitiligo

Scenario-Based Questions: Identifying Skin Abnormalities

1. Scenario: During an examination, you observe yellowing of the skin and eyes in a patient. What could this indicate?

Answer

: Yellowing of the skin and eyes is generally a sign of jaundice, often related to liver dysfunction or hemolysis. Further diagnostic tests like liver function tests are usually warranted.

2. Scenario: A patient presents with multiple small, fluid-filled blisters localized on one side of the body. What is your suspected diagnosis?

Answer

: This presentation is suggestive of herpes zoster (shingles). Antiviral treatment and symptomatic care are often recommended.

    3. Scenario: You find a pigmented lesion with irregular borders and varying colours. What is your next step?

Answer

: A pigmented lesion with irregular features is concerning for melanoma. A biopsy and further diagnostic work-up are generally required immediately.

This self-assessment is an educational tool and should not replace a thorough clinical evaluation. Always consult a healthcare professional for diagnosis and treatment.

Chapter Eighteen

Pediatric Examinations

Topics Covered:

1. **Introduction**: Understanding the unique aspects of pediatric examinations and why they differ from adult examinations.

2. **Age-Appropriate Techniques**: Tailoring the examination techniques to the developmental stage of the child.

   - Neonatal: Focus on primitive reflexes and sensory responses.

   - Infants: Observe for developmental milestones.

   - Toddlers and Preschoolers: Use of play and distraction.

   - School-age Children: Introduce educational elements to

explain procedures.

- Adolescents: Respect for privacy and autonomy.

3. **Growth and Development Assessments**: Techniques for measuring height, weight, and head circumference, and interpreting growth charts.

4. **Behavioral and Social Assessments**: Evaluating social behaviors, play, and interactions.

5. **Immunization Status**: Keeping track of the child's vaccination history.

6. **Nutritional Assessment**: Special attention to signs of malnutrition or obesity.

7. **Special Areas of Focus**:

- ENT (Ears, Nose, Throat)

- Eyesight and Hearing

- Oral Health

- Skin Conditions common in childhood, such as diaper rash or eczema

8. **Common Pediatric Conditions**: Brief overview of conditions commonly encountered in pediatric practice, such as respiratory infections, gastrointestinal issues, and childhood injuries.

Self-Assessment:

Multiple-Choice Quiz: Pediatric Examination Techniques

1. What is the most appropriate method to engage a toddler during an examination?

a) Explain the procedure in detail

b) Use of play and distraction

c) Ask the child to hold still

d) Offer a reward for cooperation

2. At what age should a child's head circumference generally stop being measured routinely?

a) 1 year

b) 2 years

c) 3 years

d) 5 years

3. Which one of the following is a common pediatric skin condition?

a) Eczema

b) Melanoma

c) Psoriasis

d) Shingles

Scenario-Based Questions:

1. Scenario: A 4-year-old child refuses to open their mouth for an oral examination. What technique could you use?

Answer

: Utilizing distraction techniques, such as asking the child to "roar like a lion," can sometimes make them more willing to open their mouth for the examination.

    2. Scenario: A teenager appears uncomfortable when their parent is in the examination room. What should you do?

Answer

: Ask the parent to step out or give the teenager the option to have part of the exam conducted privately. This respects the adolescent's need for autonomy and privacy.

This chapter serves as a resource for healthcare professionals working in pediatrics, but it is also beneficial for general practitioners and family medicine physicians who see patients of all ages. It is not a substitute for professional medical advice and clinical judgement.

Chapter Nineteen

Geriatric Examinations

Topics Covered:

1. **Introduction**: Recognizing the unique challenges and opportunities in physical examinations of older adults.

2. **Special Considerations for Older Adults**:

   - Sensory limitations: Adjustments for hearing loss, vision problems, etc.

   - Mobility issues: Examination accommodations for arthritis or other mobility challenges.

   - Cognitive assessments: Screenings for memory loss or other cognitive impairments.

3. **Polypharmacy**: Addressing the use of multiple medications

and potential interactions.

4. **Nutritional Assessments**: Identifying signs of malnutrition, dehydration, or weight loss.

5. **Functional Assessments**: Evaluating activities of daily living (ADL) and instrumental activities of daily living (IADL) capacities.

6. **Pain Management**: Assessment and documentation of chronic or acute pain.

7. **Psychosocial Factors**: Assessing the patient's living situation, social support network, and mental health.

8. **Preventive Measures**: Discuss vaccinations, screenings, and other preventative actions suited for older adults.

Self-Assessment:

Multiple-Choice Quiz: Geriatric Examination Techniques

1. What is a common issue you should know when examining an older adult?

a) Overactivity
b) Sensory limitations
c) Lack of medication
d) Excessive strength

2. Which assessment is crucial for older adults living alone?

a) ADL and IADL assessment

b) Cognitive assessment

c) Mobility assessment

d) All of the above

3. What is a critical consideration in pain management for older adults?

a) Limiting all medications to reduce side effects

b) Ignoring verbal complaints if vital signs are stable

c) Employing both pharmacological and non-pharmacological methods

d) Using the same pain scale as for younger adults

Scenario-Based Questions:

1. Scenario: An older patient has difficulty hearing your questions during the history taking. What do you do?

Answer

: Use visual aids to support your questions, or write them down if necessary. Ensure that hearing aids are functioning correctly if the patient uses them.

2. Scenario: You notice signs of potential cognitive decline during your examination. How do you proceed?

Answer

: Make a note in the patient's medical record and discuss further cognitive testing and possible referral to a specialist with the patient and their family, if appropriate.

This chapter is intended as a resource for healthcare professionals who encounter older adults in their practice. It aims to equip professionals with the knowledge and tools they need to provide high-quality care tailored to the unique needs of older adults.

Chapter Twenty

Pregnancy and Obstetrical Examinations

Topics Covered:

1. **Introduction**: The importance of specialized examination techniques in obstetrics and the unique physiological changes that occur during pregnancy.

2. **Initial Assessment**:

   - Confirming pregnancy through medical history and early symptoms

   - Discussing prenatal care plans and establishing a timetable for future visits

3. **Physical Changes in Pregnancy**:

- Cardiovascular system adjustments

- Respiratory changes

- Musculoskeletal changes

4. **Special Techniques in Pregnancy Examination**:

- Fundal height measurement

- Leopold's maneuvers

- Fetal heart rate monitoring

- Speculum and bimanual examination (when necessary and with consent)

5. **Precautions and Cautions**:

- Avoiding unnecessary radiation exposure

- Safe positioning during examinations (e.g., left lateral position)

- Awareness of signs of preeclampsia or gestational diabetes

6. **Ultrasound Evaluations**:

- Timing and purpose of different types of prenatal ultrasounds

7. **Genetic Screening and Counseling**:

○ Discussing the options, pros, and cons of genetic testing and screening during pregnancy

Self-Assessment:

Multiple-Choice Quiz: Pregnancy and Obstetrical Examinations

1. Which of the following is not commonly measured during a pregnancy examination?

a) Blood Pressure
b) Fundal Height
c) Fetal Hair Color
d) Fetal Heart Rate

2. What is one of the key cautions to take during a pregnancy examination?

a) Avoid using a stethoscope to limit stress on the fetus
b) Avoid unnecessary radiation exposure
c) Conduct the examination in a standing position
d) Avoid any kind of ultrasound

3. What is Leopold's maneuvers used for?

a) Assessing the position of the fetus
b) Measuring blood pressure
c) Confirming pregnancy
d) Screening for genetic abnormalities

Scenario-Based Questions:

1. Scenario: A pregnant patient mentions she's experiencing frequent headaches and visual disturbances. What steps should be taken?

Answer

: These may be signs of preeclampsia and require immediate attention. Check blood pressure, perform necessary lab tests, and consult with an obstetrician for further evaluation and management.

2. Scenario: During a routine examination, you notice that the fetal heart rate is irregular. What do you do?

Answer

: An irregular fetal heart rate could be a sign of distress and should be further evaluated with advanced monitoring and ultrasound. Immediate consultation with an obstetrician is advised.

This chapter serves as a comprehensive guide for healthcare professionals to understand the unique aspects and challenges of conducting physical examinations for pregnant women. It aims to provide clinicians with practical knowledge and tools for ensuring the health and well-being of both the mother and the unborn child.

Chapter Twenty-One

Medical Record Keeping

Introduction:

A ccurate and comprehensive medical record-keeping is a cornerstone of effective patient care. These records serve multiple purposes, from guiding current treatment plans to informing future medical decisions, and have legal implications. This chapter will focus on the principles of good documentation practices in the context of physical examinations and history-taking.

Objectives:

- Understand the importance of accurate and thorough medical documentation.

- Learn the standard formats and components for different types of medical records.

- Recognize the legal implications of medical record-keeping

Topics Covered:

1. **Purpose and Importance of Medical Records**:

   ○ Role in patient care, research, and legal cases

   ○ Importance for continuity of care

2. **Types of Medical Records**:

   ○ Electronic Medical Records (EMRs)

   ○ Paper Records

   ○ Specialized Records (like birth records, immunization records, etc.)

3. **Components of a Good Medical Record**:

   ○ Identifying data

   ○ Chief complaint

   ○ History of Present Illness (HPI)

   ○ Past Medical History (PMH)

   ○ Review of Systems (ROS)

   ○ Physical examination findings

- Diagnostic test results

- Treatment plans

4. Legal Implications:

- Legal requirements for record-keeping

- Handling requests for medical records

- Role of medical records in legal cases

5. Practical Tips for Effective Documentation:

- Using clear, non-ambiguous language

- Avoiding common pitfalls (e.g., illegible handwriting, incomplete sentences)

- Using standardized abbreviations

6. Technological Tools for Documentation:

- EMR software features

- Voice-to-text applications

- Secure storage solutions

Self-Assessment:

Multiple-Choice Quiz: Medical Record Keeping

1. What is NOT a standard component of an excellent medical record?

a) Identifying data

b) Social Media Profiles

c) History of Present Illness

d) Treatment plans

2. Which of the following could be a legal implication of poor medical record-keeping?

a) Loss of license

b) Increased patient satisfaction

c) Faster diagnosis

d) None of the above

3. What is one significant benefit of Electronic Medical Records (EMRs) over paper records?

a) EMRs are less secure

b) EMRs are easier to lose

c) EMRs can be easily shared among different healthcare providers

d) EMRs are more challenging to update

Scenario-Based Questions:

1. Scenario: You find an error in a patient's medical record. What should you do?

Answer

: Never alter the original entry. Make a new entry to correct the error, indicating why the correction was made, and include the date and your identification.

2. Scenario: A patient requests a copy of their medical record, but you notice it includes sensitive information that could be harmful if misinterpreted. How do you proceed?

Answer

: Consult the legal guidelines in your jurisdiction and discuss the sensitive nature of the information with the patient. It's generally the patient's right to access their records, but professional discretion can be used.

By understanding the significance and legal implications of medical documentation, healthcare professionals can improve their practice, minimize risks, and, ultimately, provide better patient care.

Chapter Twenty-Two

Correlating History and Physical Findings to Formulate a Differential Diagnosis

Introduction:

C ombining insights from a patient's history and physical examination is a crucial step in arriving at a diagnosis. This chapter aims to guide healthcare practitioners in how to synthesize these individual elements into a cohesive and meaningful framework, known as the differential diagnosis.

Objectives:

- Develop the skill of correlating medical history and physical examination findings.

- Understand the process of formulating a differential diagnosis.

- Learn techniques for refining the list of potential diagnoses to reach the most accurate conclusion.

Topics Covered:

1. The Art of Correlation:

- Using history to guide the physical examination and vice versa

- Confirmatory and disconfirmatory signs and symptoms

2. Steps in Formulating a Differential Diagnosis:

- Listing possible diagnoses based on initial findings

- Ordering them based on likelihood

- Considering worst-case scenarios

3. Use of Diagnostic Tests:

- When and how to employ additional diagnostic tests to narrow down the differential diagnosis

- Understanding the limitations and pitfalls of various diagnostic tests

4. Interdisciplinary Consultations:

- When to seek advice from specialists

- How to interpret consultation notes and incorporate them into the differential diagnosis

5. Clinical Reasoning Tools:

- Diagnostic algorithms

- Bayesian reasoning

- Decision trees

6. Case Studies:

- Real-world examples illustrating the process of formulating a differential diagnosis

Self-Assessment:

Multiple-Choice Quiz: Formulating a Differential Diagnosis

1. Which is NOT a step in formulating a differential diagnosis?

a) Listing all possible diagnoses based on history and physical findings

b) Ignoring worst-case scenarios to alleviate patient anxiety

c) Ordering diagnoses based on likelihood

d) Employing additional diagnostic tests to narrow down the list

   2. What should be done when two or more potential diagnoses have similar likelihood?

a) Choose the one that is easier to treat

b) Seek interdisciplinary consultation

c) Ignore the less severe one

d) All of the above

Scenario-Based Questions:

   1. Scenario: Your patient presents with acute abdominal pain. After collecting the history and performing a physical exam, you suspect it might be either appendicitis or a kidney stone. What should be your next step?

Answer

: Employ additional diagnostic tests such as ultrasound or CT scan to differentiate between the two. If still uncertain, consider consulting a specialist in gastroenterology or nephrology.

   2. Scenario: You are faced with a case where the patient's symptoms don't clearly point to any of the likely diagnoses. What approach should you take?

Answer

: Revisit the patient's history and re-evaluate your physical exam findings. If necessary, consult with specialists and consider running more diagnostic tests to cover a broader range of possibilities.

Correlating history and physical findings is both an art and a science. The quality of this correlation often determines how quickly and accurately a healthcare provider can identify the underlying issue. Developing these skills will not only help in improving patient outcomes but also contribute to a more efficient and effective healthcare system.

Chapter Twenty-Three

Common Diagnostic Tests

T his chapter provides an overview of common diagnostic tests used in medical practice. Understanding the purposes of these tests and their indications is essential for healthcare professionals to make informed decisions regarding patient care and diagnosis.

Objectives:

- Familiarize healthcare professionals with a range of common diagnostic tests.

- Understand the purposes of these tests and when they should be used.

- Enhance knowledge of which medical conditions or issues each test can help diagnose or monitor.

Topics Covered:

1. Complete Blood Count (CBC):

○ Purpose: Assess overall health and detect a variety of disorders, such as anemia and infection.

○ Indications: Unexplained fever, fatigue, weakness, or bruising; monitoring certain medical conditions.

2. Comprehensive Metabolic Panel (CMP):

○ Purpose: Evaluate organ function, electrolyte balance, and glucose levels.

○ Indications: To assess overall health, screen for certain conditions, or monitor existing medical conditions.

3. X-Ray Imaging:

○ Purpose: Visualize bones, joints, and some soft tissues for diagnosing fractures, infections, and other conditions.

○ Indications: Suspected bone fractures, lung infections, and joint issues.

4. Computed Tomography (CT) Scan:

○ Purpose: Produce detailed cross-sectional images of the body for diagnosing a wide range of conditions.

○ Indications: Evaluation of head injuries, abdominal

pain, and detection of tumors.

5. Magnetic Resonance Imaging (MRI):

- Purpose: Provide detailed images of soft tissues and organs for diagnosing various medical conditions.

- Indications: Detecting brain and spinal cord abnormalities, evaluating joints, and assessing soft tissue structures.

6. Electrocardiogram (ECG or EKG):

- Purpose: Record the heart's electrical activity to diagnose heart-related issues.

- Indications: Chest pain, palpitations, and assessing heart function.

7. Biopsy:

- Purpose: Obtain tissue samples for laboratory analysis to diagnose or rule out cancer and other diseases.

- Indications: Suspicious lumps or lesions, abnormal imaging findings.

8. Endoscopy:

- Purpose: Visualize the inside of organs or structures using a flexible tube with a camera.

- Indications: Gastrointestinal issues, assessment of the respiratory tract, and detection of abnormalities.

Self-Assessment:

Multiple-Choice Quiz: Diagnostic Test Purposes and Indications

1. What is the primary purpose of a Complete Blood Count (CBC)?

a) To evaluate organ function
b) To visualize soft tissues
c) To assess overall health and detect disorders
d) To record the heart's electrical activity

2. When might an Electrocardiogram (ECG or EKG) typically be used?

a) To assess overall health
b) To diagnose bone fractures
c) To record brain activity
d) To diagnose heart-related issues

Scenario-Based Questions:

1. Scenario: A patient presents with unexplained fatigue and weakness. Which diagnostic test would be most appropriate, and why?

Answer
: A Complete Blood Count (CBC) would be appropriate to assess overall health and detect any disorders, such as anemia or infection, which might be causing the fatigue and weakness.

2. Scenario: A patient experiences severe abdominal pain. What diagnostic imaging test might help diagnose the issue, and what could it potentially detect?

Answer

: A Computed Tomography (CT) scan may be used to visualize the abdominal area and detect conditions such as appendicitis, kidney stones, or tumors.

Understanding the purposes and indications of common diagnostic tests is fundamental for healthcare professionals in providing effective patient care. This knowledge assists in making informed decisions about which tests are appropriate for a given clinical scenario.

Chapter Twenty-Four

Summary of Key Points

1. **Physical Examination and History Taking**:

   - Physical examination and history taking are fundamental components of medical practice.

   - The history-taking process involves gathering information about a patient's medical history, including past illnesses, family history, and current symptoms.

   - The physical examination involves the systematic assessment of a patient's body to identify signs of illness or injury.

2. Importance of Accuracy:

- Accurate and thorough history taking and physical examination are crucial for making accurate diagnoses and treatment decisions.

- Healthcare professionals must actively listen to patients, ask open-ended questions, and use effective communication skills.

3. Documentation:

- Proper documentation of patient information, findings, and diagnoses is essential for continuity of care and legal purposes.

- Medical records should include identifying data, chief complaint, history of present illness, past medical history, review of systems, physical examination findings, and treatment plans.

4. Professionalism and Ethics:

- Healthcare professionals must adhere to ethical principles, including patient privacy and informed consent.

- Building rapport and practicing basic communication skills are key to effective patient interactions.

5. Differential Diagnosis:

- Correlating history and physical examination findings is crucial for formulating a differential diagnosis.

- The differential diagnosis is a list of potential diagnoses ranked by likelihood.

6. Diagnostic Testing:

- Diagnostic tests, such as blood tests, imaging, and biopsies, play a vital role in confirming or ruling out diagnoses.

- The selection of diagnostic tests should be based on clinical indications, risk vs. benefit analysis, and patient preferences.

7. Future Trends:

- Future trends in physical examination and history taking may include the integration of technology, such as telemedicine and wearable devices, to enhance data collection.

- AI-driven tools may assist healthcare professionals in data analysis and decision-making.

- Patient-centered care and shared decision-making are expected to become even more prominent in medical practice.

8. Continuing Education:

- Healthcare professionals should stay updated with advances in medical practice and continue their education to provide the best possible care to patients.

Future Trends in Physical Examination and History Taking

1. Telemedicine and Remote Monitoring:

- Telemedicine is expected to continue growing, allowing healthcare professionals to conduct remote history taking and consultations.

- Wearable devices and remote monitoring tools may provide real-time health data for better assessment.

2. Artificial Intelligence (AI):

- AI-driven algorithms and machine learning may assist in pattern recognition and data analysis during history taking and physical examination.

- AI can provide decision support to healthcare professionals.

3. Patient-Centered Care:

- The emphasis on patient-centered care is likely to increase, with a focus on involving patients in their own healthcare decisions.

- Shared decision-making and patient empowerment will play a significant role.

4. Genomics and Personalized Medicine:

○ Advances in genomics may lead to more personalized history taking and treatment plans, considering an individual's genetic profile.

5. Interdisciplinary Collaboration:

○ Collaboration between healthcare professionals from different specialties is expected to enhance the comprehensive assessment of patients.

6. Continuous Learning:

○ Healthcare professionals will need to engage in continuous learning to stay updated with evolving practices, technologies, and ethical considerations.

The future of physical examination and history taking is likely to be shaped by technological advancements, patient-centered approaches, and a commitment to providing high-quality, personalized care. Healthcare professionals must adapt to these changes while upholding ethical principles and maintaining their commitment to accuracy and professionalism.

Chapter Twenty-Five

Appendices

Appendix A: Sample Medical History Form

- A template for a comprehensive medical history form that can be used in clinical practice.

Appendix B: Physical Examination Checklist

- A checklist outlining the key components of a thorough physical examination, organized by body systems.

Appendix C: Common Medical Abbreviations

- A list of frequently used medical abbreviations and their meanings to assist in understanding medical documentation.

Appendix D: Informed Consent Template

- A sample informed consent template that healthcare professionals can use when obtaining patient consent for procedures or treatments.

Appendix E: Differential Diagnosis Worksheet

- A worksheet to assist in formulating a differential diagnosis, with space to list potential diagnoses and rank them by likelihood.

Appendix F: Diagnostic Test Reference Guide

- An overview of common diagnostic tests, including their purposes, indications, and potential findings.

Appendix G: Resources for Continuing Education

- A list of reputable sources, websites, and organizations that offer educational resources and courses for healthcare professionals to stay updated in their field.

Appendix H: Glossary of Medical Terms

- A glossary containing definitions of medical terminology used throughout the book for quick reference.

Appendix I: References

- A list of academic and professional references used to compile the information in the book for readers interested in further research and reading.

These appendices provide valuable tools and resources to complement the information presented in the book. They serve as practical references for healthcare professionals in their clinical practice and ongoing education.

Chapter Twenty-Six

Sample Template: Patient Medical History Form

P atient Information:

- N   a   m   e   :

  _____

- **Date of Birth**: //_____

- **Gender**: [ ] Male [ ] Female [ ] Other

- A   d   d   r   e   s   s   :

  _____

- **Phone Number**: _____

- E   m   a   i   l   :

  _____

Emergency Contact:
- N   a   m   e   :

  _____

- R   e   l   a   t   i   o   n   s   h   i   p   :

  _____

- Phone Number: _____

Primary Care Physician:
- N   a   m   e   :

  _____

- Phone Number: _____

Insurance Information:
- Primary   Insurance:

  _____

- Policy   Number:

  _____

- Secondary   Insurance:

  _____

- Policy   Number:

  _____

Medical History:

1. Current Medications:
- Please list all medications, including prescription, over-the-counter, and supplements, that you are currently taking.

2. Allergies:

- List any allergies you have, including medications, foods, environmental allergens, and latex.

3. Past Medical History:

- Please check any conditions you have been diagnosed with or have a history of:

[ ] High Blood Pressure [ ] Heart Disease [ ] Diabetes [ ] Asthma
[ ] Cancer [ ] Arthritis [ ] Kidney Disease [ ] Stroke
[ ] Epilepsy [ ] Thyroid Disorder [ ] Chronic Obstructive Pulmonary Disease (COPD)
[   ]   Other   (please   specify):

_____

4. Surgical History:

- List any past surgeries, including dates and reasons:

5. Family Medical History:

- Please note any significant medical conditions in your immediate family (parents, siblings, children):

6. Social History:

- Smoker [ ] Non-Smoker [ ] Former Smoker (If yes, please specify the number of years smoked)

- Alcohol Use (If yes, please specify frequency and quantity)

- Recreational Drug Use (If yes, please specify type and frequency)

- Exercise Habits (If yes, please specify type and frequency)

7. Women Only:

- Pregnant [ ] Breastfeeding [ ] Menstrual History (Please specify any issues)

- Hysterectomy [ ] Menopause [ ] Birth Control Method (If applicable)

8. Additional Information:

- Is there any other information or medical history you believe is important for your healthcare provider to know?

Signature:

I certify that the information provided is accurate and complete to the best of my knowledge.

Patient's Signature: _____

Date: //_____

Please note that this is a sample template and can be modified to suit the specific needs of your healthcare practice. It's important to ensure that patients fill out the form accurately, as it serves as a crucial part of their medical record.

Chapter
Twenty-Seven

Physical
Examination
Checklist

Patient Information:

- N a m e :

  _____

- Date of Birth: //_____

- Date of Examination: //_____

- Medical Record Number:

  _____

General Appearance:
- Alert and oriented

- Well-nourished

- Well-hydrated

- Comfortable at rest

- Cachectic or wasted appearance

- Signs of distress or discomfort

Vital Signs:
- Temperature: _____°F/°C

- Blood Pressure: / mmHg

- Heart Rate: _____ bpm

- Respiratory Rate: _____ breaths/min

- Oxygen Saturation: _____%

- Pain Assessment: _____/10 (if applicable)

Head and Neck:
- Inspection of scalp and hair

- Examination of eyes (pupils, sclera, conjunctiva)

- Examination of ears (external and internal)

- Examination of nose (nares, mucosa)

- Examination of throat and oral cavity

- Palpation of lymph nodes

Chest and Lungs:

- Inspection of chest symmetry and respiratory effort

- Palpation of chest for tenderness or masses

- Percussion of lung fields

- Auscultation of lung sounds (breath sounds, adventitious sounds)

Cardiovascular System:

- Inspection and palpation of precordium (chest wall)

- Palpation of apical pulse

- Auscultation of heart sounds (S1, S2, additional sounds)

- Assessment of peripheral pulses (radial, femoral, pedal, etc.)

- Assessment of edema (if applicable)

Abdomen:

- Inspection of abdominal contour and symmetry

- Auscultation of bowel sounds

- Palpation of abdomen (tenderness, masses)

- Percussion of abdominal quadrants

- Examination of liver and spleen (if indicated)

- Assessment of hernias (if applicable)

Musculoskeletal System:

- Inspection of posture and gait

- Palpation of joints (range of motion, tenderness)

- Assessment of muscle strength

- Evaluation of spine (curvature, alignment)

- Examination of extremities (edema, pulses, skin)

Neurological System:

- Assessment of mental status (orientation, memory)

- Assessment of cranial nerves (if indicated)

- Evaluation of motor function (strength, coordination)

- Examination of sensation (light touch, pain, temperature)

- Reflex testing (deep tendon reflexes)

- Assessment of gait and balance

Skin and Integumentary System:

- Inspection of skin color, texture, and lesions

- Assessment of skin turgor

- Examination of nails (color, shape)

- Assessment of hair distribution

- Palpation of lymph nodes (if not assessed earlier)

Genital and Rectal Examination (if indicated):

- Examination of external genitalia (male/female)

- Speculum examination (female)

- Digital rectal examination (if indicated)

Additional Notes and Findings:

-

-

-

Plan and Recommendations:

-

-

-

Signature:

I certify that I have completed a thorough physical examination of the patient in accordance with the checklist.

Healthcare   Provider's   Signature:

_____ **Date:** //_____

Please note that this is a sample template and can be customized to suit specific clinical settings and preferences. Healthcare providers should perform a thorough physical examination based on the patient's medical history and presenting complaints. The checklist serves as a documentation tool to ensure that all relevant aspects of the examination have been addressed.

Chapter Twenty-Eight

Common Medical Abbrevations

A

- **ABG**: Arterial Blood Gas

- **ACL**: Anterior Cruciate Ligament

- **ADL**: Activities of Daily Living

- **AFib**: Atrial Fibrillation

- **AIDS**: Acquired Immunodeficiency Syndrome

- **A&P**: Assessment and Plan

- **ASAP**: As Soon As Possible

B

- **BID**: Twice a Day (from Latin "bis in die")

- **BP**: Blood Pressure

- **BPM**: Beats Per Minute

- **BUN**: Blood Urea Nitrogen

C

- **CBC**: Complete Blood Count

- **CC**: Chief Complaint

- **CNS**: Central Nervous System

- **COPD**: Chronic Obstructive Pulmonary Disease

- **CP**: Chest Pain

- **CRP**: C-Reactive Protein

- **CSF**: Cerebrospinal Fluid

- **CVA**: Cerebrovascular Accident (Stroke)

D

- **DNR**: Do Not Resuscitate

- **DVT**: Deep Vein Thrombosis

E

- **ECG/EKG**: Electrocardiogram

- **ENT**: Ear, Nose, and Throat

- **ER**: Emergency Room

- **ESR**: Erythrocyte Sedimentation Rate

F

- **FBS**: Fasting Blood Sugar

- **FUO**: Fever of Unknown Origin

H

- **H&P**: History and Physical

- **HR**: Heart Rate

- **HTN**: Hypertension (High Blood Pressure)

I

- **ICU**: Intensive Care Unit

- **IV**: Intravenous

L

- **LMP**: Last Menstrual Period

- **LOS**: Length of Stay

N

- **NPO**: Nothing by Mouth (from Latin "nil per os")

O

- **OB/GYN**: Obstetrics and Gynecology

- **OTC**: Over-the-Counter

P

- **PCP**: Primary Care Physician

- **PRN**: As Needed (from Latin "pro re nata")

- **PT**: Physical Therapy

- **PTT**: Partial Thromboplastin Time

Q

- **QD**: Once a Day (from Latin "quaque die")

- **QID**: Four Times a Day (from Latin "quater in die")

R

- **ROM**: Range of Motion

- **Rx**: Prescription

S

- **SOB**: Shortness of Breath

- **STAT**: Immediately (from Latin "statim")

T

- **TID**: Three Times a Day (from Latin "ter in die")

U

- **UTI**: Urinary Tract Infection

W

- **WBC**: White Blood Cell Count

Please note that medical abbreviations can vary, and it's essential to clarify their meaning if there is any uncertainty. Additionally, some abbreviations may have different meanings in different medical contexts, so context is important for accurate interpretation.

Informed Consent for Medical Procedure or Treatment

P atient Information:

- Patient's   Name:

  _____

- Date of Birth: //_____

- Medical   Record   Number:

- **P r o c e d u r e / T r e a t m e n t :**

- **Date of Procedure/Treatment: //_____**

Purpose and Description:

I, [Patient's Name], hereby grant my informed consent for the performance of the following medical procedure/treatment, as described below:

Procedure/Treatment Description:

[Provide a clear and concise description of the procedure or treatment, including its purpose, expected benefits, risks, alternatives, and any special instructions or preparations.]

Purpose:

[Explain the medical necessity or intended outcome of the procedure or treatment.]

Benefits:

[Describe the potential benefits or expected outcomes of the procedure or treatment.]

Risks:

[Outline any potential risks, complications, or side effects associated with the procedure or treatment.]

Alternatives:

[Discuss alternative treatments or options available and their advantages and disadvantages.]

Special Instructions/Preparations:

[Include any specific instructions or preparations the patient should follow before the procedure or treatment.]

Consent:

I have had the opportunity to discuss the procedure/treatment described above with my healthcare provider, [Provider's Name], who has answered my questions to my satisfaction. I understand the purpose, benefits, and risks of the procedure/treatment, as well as the alternatives. I have been informed of the expected outcome and any special instructions or preparations required.

I hereby voluntarily consent to undergo the described procedure/treatment, understanding that it may involve certain risks and potential complications. I understand that no guarantees or assurances have been made regarding the outcome, as medical outcomes can vary from person to person.

Patient's Signature: _____

Date: //_____

Witness (if applicable):

I, [Witness's Name], certify that I have witnessed the patient's signature on this informed consent form and that the patient appears to have made an informed and voluntary decision.

Witness's Signature: _____

Date: //_____

Please note that this is a sample template and should be customized to fit the specific procedure or treatment, as well as any legal and institutional requirements. It's crucial to provide patients with clear and comprehensive information and to ensure that they have the opportunity to ask questions and fully understand the implications of the procedure or treatment before giving their informed consent. Additionally, some procedures may require multiple forms or additional documentation, depending on the complexity and nature of the medical intervention.

Chapter Thirty

Differential Diagnosis Worksheet

P atient Information:
- **Patient's** **Name:**

  _____

- **Date of Birth:** //_____

- **Date of Evaluation:** //_____

- **Medical** **Record** **Number:**

  _____

Chief Complaint:

[Describe the patient's main symptom or complaint.]

Presenting Symptoms and Findings:

[List all relevant symptoms, physical findings, and laboratory results.]

Potential Diagnoses:

[Based on the patient's presentation, list potential diagnoses that need to be considered.]

1. Diagnosis:

_____

- Likelihood: [ ] High [ ] Moderate [ ] Low

- Rationale:

_____

2. Diagnosis:

_____

- Likelihood: [ ] High [ ] Moderate [ ] Low

- Rationale:

_____

3. Diagnosis:

_____

- Likelihood: [ ] High [ ] Moderate [ ] Low

- Rationale:

_____

4. Diagnosis:

_____

- Likelihood: [ ] High [ ] Moderate [ ] Low

- Rationale:

_____

5. D   i   a   g   n   o   s   i   s   :

_____

    ◦ Likelihood: [ ] High [ ] Moderate [ ] Low

    ◦ R   a   t   i   o   n   a   l   e   :

_____

Additional Diagnostic Tests or Evaluations Needed:
[List any additional tests, imaging studies, or consultations required
to confirm or rule out potential diagnoses.]

    1. T   e   s   t   /   S   t   u   d   y   :

_____

    ◦ R   a   t   i   o   n   a   l   e   :

_____

    2. T   e   s   t   /   S   t   u   d   y   :

_____

    ◦ R   a   t   i   o   n   a   l   e   :

_____

    3. T   e   s   t   /   S   t   u   d   y   :

_____

    ◦ R   a   t   i   o   n   a   l   e   :

_____

Treatment and Management Plan:
[Outline initial treatment and management strategies based on the
most likely diagnosis, if identified.]

    1. T r e a t m e n t / M a n a g e m e n t :

○ R a t i o n a l e :

Follow-Up Plan:

[Specify when the patient should return for a follow-up evaluation, re-assessment, or further tests.]

Patient and Family Education:

[Provide information and instructions for the patient and their family regarding the condition and its management.]

Provider's Signature: _____

Date: //_____

This worksheet is a sample template and should be customized to fit the specific clinical situation. Differential diagnosis is a critical process in healthcare, and organizing potential diagnoses and their likelihoods can help guide further evaluation and treatment decisions. It's essential to involve the patient in the decision-making process and to consider their preferences and values when determining the best course of action.

Chapter Thirty-One

Diagnostic Test Reference Guide

Test Name: [Name of Diagnostic Test]

Purpose:

- [Briefly describe the primary purpose or objective of the test.]

Indications:

- [List the clinical scenarios or conditions for which the test is commonly ordered.]

Procedure:

- [Provide a brief overview of how the test is conducted, including any special preparations or patient instructions.]

Normal Range/Findings:

- [Specify the normal range or findings expected in a healthy individual.]

Abnormal Findings:

- [Describe the potential abnormal findings or results that may indicate a medical condition.]

Interpretation:

- [Explain how healthcare providers typically interpret the results.]

Common Uses:

- [Provide examples of common medical conditions or situations where the test is valuable.]

Risks and Considerations:

- [Highlight any potential risks, contraindications, or special considerations associated with the test.]

Follow-Up:

- [Explain what steps may follow if the test results are abnormal or inconclusive.]

Examples:

- [Include specific medical conditions or scenarios where the test is frequently used.]

Please note that this is a sample template, and the content should be customized to reflect the specific diagnostic tests used in your healthcare practice. Additionally, it's essential to stay updated with the latest guidelines and recommendations for each diagnostic test as the field of medicine continually evolves. Healthcare providers should use this reference guide to aid in patient education and communication about diagnostic testing.

Chapter Thirty-Two

Resources for Continuing Education

R eputable sources, websites, and organizations that offer educational resources and courses for healthcare professionals to stay updated in their field:

1. **Medscape Education**: Medscape offers various free continuing medical education (CME) courses, articles, and resources covering multiple medical specialties.

Website:

Medscape Education

2. **Coursera**: Coursera partners with top universities and institutions to provide online courses, including those related to healthcare and medicine. Many systems offer certificates upon completion.

Website:

Coursera

3. **edX**: Similar to Coursera, edX collaborates with universities to offer online courses. They provide both free and paid courses, with options for professional certifications.

Website:

edX

4. **Khan Academy**: Khan Academy offers free online courses and tutorials covering various healthcare topics, including anatomy, physiology, and medicine.

Website:

Khan Academy Medicine

5. **American Medical Association (AMA)**: The AMA offers CME opportunities and resources for physicians and healthcare professionals, including journals and events.

Website:

AMA Continuing Medical Education

6. **National Institutes of Health (NIH) Training and Events**: NIH provides various training and educational opportunities for healthcare professionals, researchers, and students.

Website:

NIH Training

7. **UpToDate**: UpToDate offers evidence-based clinical decision support resources, including CME credits for reading and using their content.

Website:

UpToDate

8. **Harvard Medical School Online Learning**: Harvard Medical School offers online courses and programs for healthcare professionals covering various medical topics.

Website:

Harvard Online Learning

9. **American Nurses Credentialing Center (ANCC)**: ANCC provides continuing education resources and opportunities for nurses and nurse practitioners.

Website:

ANCC Continuing Education

10. **Online MedEd**: Online MedEd offers free and paid educational resources, including video lectures and study tools, primarily focused on medical students and residents.

Website:

Online MedEd

11. **JAMA Network CME**: The Journal of the American Medical Association (JAMA) offers CME activities and resources for healthcare professionals.

Website:

JAMA Network CME

12. **Cleveland Clinic Center for Continuing Education**: The Cleveland Clinic offers a variety of CME opportunities and resources for healthcare providers.

Website:

Cleveland Clinic CME

13. **Continuing Dental Education Online (CDEWorld)**: CDEWorld provides dental professionals with online dental

continuing education courses and resources.

Website:

CDEWorld

Please note that the availability and content of educational resources may change over time, so it's a good practice to verify the most up-to-date information on these websites. Additionally, some resources may require registration or payment for specific courses or certifications.

Chapter
Thirty-Three

Glossary of
Medical Terms

A **•Abdomen**: The area of the body located between the chest and the pelvis, containing organs such as the stomach, liver, and intestines.

- **Adverse Reaction**: An unintended and harmful response to a medication or medical treatment.

- **Anatomy**: The study of the structure and organization of the body and its organs.

- **Antibiotic**: A type of medication used to treat bacterial infections.

- **Antigen**: A substance that can trigger an immune response in the body.

B

- **Blood Pressure**: The force of blood against the walls of the arteries. It is measured in millimeters of mercury (mm Hg) and consists of systolic and diastolic pressures.

- **Bronchitis**: Inflammation of the bronchial tubes, often causing coughing and difficulty breathing.

C

- **Cardiology**: The medical specialty focused on the study and treatment of heart-related conditions.

- **Chronic**: A condition or disease that persists over a long period or is recurrent.

- **Clinical Trial**: A research study involving human participants to evaluate the safety and effectiveness of medical interventions.

- **Colonoscopy**: A medical procedure used to examine the inside of the colon (large intestine) using a flexible tube with a camera.

- **Computed Tomography (CT)**: A diagnostic imaging technique that uses X-rays to create cross-sectional images of the body.

- **Cytology**: The study of cells and their structure, function, and abnormalities.

D

- **Diagnosis**: The identification of a disease or condition based on its signs, symptoms, and medical tests.

- **Dietitian**: A healthcare professional trained in nutrition and dietary management.

- **Disease**: A deviation from normal health or the functioning of the body that impairs its proper functioning.

E

- **Electrocardiogram (ECG or EKG)**: A test that records the electrical activity of the heart to diagnose heart conditions.

- **Emergency Medicine**: A medical specialty focused on the treatment of acute and life-threatening conditions.

- **Endoscopy**: A medical procedure using a thin, flexible tube with a camera to view the interior of organs or cavities.

- **Epidemiology**: The study of the distribution and determinants of diseases in populations.

- **Examination**: A systematic and detailed assessment of a patient's body or specific organ systems by a healthcare professional.

F

- **Family History**: A record of a person's family members and their medical conditions, often used to assess genetic risk factors.

- **Fever**: Elevated body temperature, often a sign of an underlying infection or inflammation.

- **Fracture**: A break or crack in a bone.

G

- **Gastroenterology**: The medical specialty focused on the study and treatment of digestive system disorders.

- **Genetics**: The study of genes, heredity, and genetic variations.

- **Geriatrics**: The medical specialty focused on the care of elderly individuals.

H

- **Hematology**: The medical specialty focused on the study and treatment of blood disorders.

- **Hypertension**: High blood pressure, a condition that can increase the risk of cardiovascular disease.

- **Hygiene**: Practices and measures to maintain cleanliness and prevent the spread of disease.

I

- **Immunization**: The process of introducing a vaccine into the body to stimulate the immune system and provide protection against specific diseases.

- **Infection**: The invasion and multiplication of harmful microorganisms, such as bacteria or viruses, in the body.

- **Inflammation**: A localized response to tissue injury or infection, often characterized by redness, swelling, pain, and heat.

J

- **Jaundice**: A yellowing of the skin and eyes due to the accumulation of bilirubin in the body, often indicating liver or bile duct problems.

K

- **Kidneys**: Pair of organs responsible for filtering waste products from the blood and regulating fluid balance.

L

- **Lungs**: Organs responsible for respiration, where oxygen is taken in and carbon dioxide is expelled.

- **Lymphatic System**: A network of vessels and nodes that transport lymph and play a role in the immune system.

M

- **Magnetic Resonance Imaging (MRI)**: A diagnostic imaging technique that uses strong magnets and radio waves to create detailed images of the body.

- **Medication**: A substance used to treat, prevent, or manage medical conditions.

- **Microbiology**: The study of microorganisms, including bacteria, viruses, and fungi.

N

- **Neurology**: The medical specialty focused on the study and treatment of neurological disorders.

- **Nutrition**: The process of obtaining and using food for growth, development, and overall health.

O

- **Obstetrics**: The medical specialty focused on pregnancy, childbirth, and the care of women during and after pregnancy.

- **Oncology**: The medical specialty focused on the study and treatment of cancer.

- **Ophthalmology**: The medical specialty focused on the study and treatment of eye disorders.

P

- **Pathology**: The study of diseases and the changes they cause in tissues and organs.

- **Pharmacy**: The profession and practice of preparing and dispensing medications.

- **Physiology**: The study of the normal functions of living organisms and their parts.

- **Psychiatry**: The medical specialty focused on the study and treatment of mental disorders.

Q

- **Quality of Life**: A measure of an individual's overall well-being and satisfaction with life, often used in healthcare assessments.

R

- **Radiology**: The medical specialty focused on diagnostic imaging techniques, such as X-rays and CT scans.

- **Respiration**: The process of breathing, involving the exchange of oxygen and carbon dioxide in the body.

- **Rheumatology**: The medical specialty focused on the study and treatment of autoimmune and musculoskeletal disorders.

S

- **Surgery**: Medical procedures involving manual or instrumental techniques to treat diseases, injuries, or conditions.

- **Symptom**: A subjective indication of a disease or condition reported by a patient.

T

- **Therapy**: Medical treatment or intervention aimed at improving a patient's health or well-being.

- **Toxicology**: The study of the adverse effects of chemicals or substances on living organisms.

U

- **Ultrasound**: A diagnostic imaging technique that uses high-frequency sound waves to create images of the body's internal structures.

- **Urology**: The medical specialty focused on the study and treatment of urinary and male reproductive system disorders.

V

- **Vaccination**: The administration of a vaccine to stimulate the immune system and provide protection against specific diseases.

- **Virus**: A small infectious agent that can replicate only within the living cells of a host organism.

W

- **Wellness**: A state of overall health and well-being, often encompassing physical, mental, and social aspects.

- **X-ray**: A form of electromagnetic radiation used in diagnostic imaging to visualize internal structures of the body.

Z

- **Zoonosis**: An infectious disease that can be transmitted from animals to humans.

Please note that this glossary is a sample and can be expanded upon with additional medical terms and definitions relevant to your book's content. It can serve as a useful reference tool for readers who may encounter unfamiliar medical terminology while reading your book.

Chapter Thirty-Four

Comprehensive Physical Examination Checklist:

U se this checklist as a guide for performing a thorough physical examination. Adapt it to the specific needs of your book and target audience.

1. **General Survey**

   - Observe the patient's overall appearance, posture, and level of distress.

   - Assess vital signs: temperature, blood pressure, heart rate, respiratory rate, and oxygen saturation.

2. **Head and Neck Examination**

- Inspect the head for symmetry, hair distribution, and scalp abnormalities.

- Examine the eyes, including visual acuity, pupil size and reaction, and fundoscopy.

- Evaluate the ears, including otoscopic examination.

- Inspect the nose and assess for any nasal abnormalities.

- Examine the mouth and throat, including oral mucosa, tonsils, and pharynx.

3. Chest and Lungs Examination

- Inspect the chest for symmetry and deformities.

- Palpate for chest expansion and tenderness.

- Auscultate lung sounds in multiple regions of the chest.

4. Cardiovascular Examination

- Palpate peripheral pulses, including carotid, brachial, radial, femoral, popliteal, and dorsalis pedis.

- Auscultate heart sounds in various areas, including the aortic, pulmonic, tricuspid, and mitral areas.

5. Abdominal Examination

- Inspect the abdomen for any masses, scars, or abdominal distension.

- Auscultate bowel sounds in all quadrants.

○ Palpate the abdomen for tenderness and organ enlargement.

6. Neurological Examination

○ Assess cranial nerves, including motor and sensory function.

○ Evaluate muscle strength and tone.

○ Test reflexes and coordination.

7. Musculoskeletal Examination

○ Examine a joint range of motion.

○ Evaluate muscle strength.

○ Check for deformities or abnormalities.

8. Skin and Dermatological Examination

○ Inspect the skin for colour, texture, lesions, and rashes.

○ Assess for any signs of skin abnormalities or infections.

9. Genitourinary Examination

○ Assess the genitalia for any abnormalities or lesions.

○ Perform a pelvic examination for female patients if indicated.

Comprehensive History-Taking Checklist:

Use this checklist to guide the process of obtaining a comprehensive medical history from the patient.

1. Identifying Data and Chief Complaints

- Record the patient's demographic information.

- Identify the reason for the patient's visit or chief complaint.

2. History of Present Illness (HPI)

- Gather a detailed account of the current illness or condition.

- Document the onset, duration, location, severity, and associated symptoms.

3. Past Medical History (PMH)

- Record previous illnesses, surgeries, and hospitalizations.

- Document any chronic medical conditions and their management.

4. Family History

- Obtain information about medical conditions that run in the patient's family.

5. Social History

- Explore the patient's lifestyle, including habits, occupation, and social support.

6. Medication History

○ Document all current medications, including prescription and over-the-counter drugs.

7. Allergies

○ Ask about any known allergies to medications or substances.

8. Review of Systems (ROS)

○ Systematically inquire about symptoms related to various body systems.

These checklists can serve as valuable tools for healthcare professionals and readers interested in learning how to conduct thorough physical examinations and gather comprehensive medical histories. You can customize and expand upon these checklists to suit the specific needs of your book.

Chapter Thirty-Five

Common Reference Charts for Normal Values

V **ital Signs:**

1. **Temperature:** Normal body temperature ranges by age:

   ○ Adults: 97.8°F to 99.1°F (36.5°C to 37.3°C)

   ○ Children: 97.8°F to 99.1°F (36.5°C to 37.3°C)

   ○ Infants: 97.8°F to 99.1°F (36.5°C to 37.3°C)

2. **Blood Pressure:** Normal blood pressure values:

   ○ Systolic (top number): Less than 120 mm Hg

○ Diastolic (bottom number): Less than 80 mm Hg

3. **Heart Rate (Pulse):** Normal heart rate ranges by age:

○ Adults: 60 to 100 beats per minute

○ Children: 70 to 120 beats per minute

○ Infants: 100 to 160 beats per minute

4. **Respiratory Rate:** Normal respiratory rate ranges by age:

○ Adults: 12 to 20 breaths per minute

○ Children: 20 to 30 breaths per minute

○ Infants: 30 to 60 breaths per minute

5. **Oxygen Saturation (SpO2):** Normal oxygen saturation levels:

○ 95% to 100%

Laboratory Values:
1. **Complete Blood Count (CBC):**

○ Hemoglobin (Hb): Adult male: 13.8 to 17.2 g/dL; Adult female: 12.1 to 15.1 g/dL

○ Hematocrit (Hct): Adult male: 38.3% to 48.6%; Adult female: 35.5% to 44.9%

○ White Blood Cell Count (WBC): 4,500 to 11,000 cells/mm^3

○ Platelet Count (Plt): 150,000 to 450,000/mm^3

2. Blood Glucose (Fasting):

○ Average fasting blood glucose level: 70 to 99 mg/dL

3. Cholesterol (Total):

○ Desirable total cholesterol level: Less than 200 mg/dL

4. Serum Electrolytes:

○ Sodium (Na+): 135 to 145 mEq/L

○ Potassium (K+): 3.5 to 5.0 mEq/L

○ Calcium (Ca2+): 8.5 to 10.5 mg/dL

5. Renal Function:

○ Creatinine (Cr): Normal range varies by age, sex, and muscle mass.

○ Blood Urea Nitrogen (BUN): 7 to 20 mg/dL

Other Parameters:
1. Body Mass Index (BMI): BMI categories:

○ Underweight: BMI less than 18.5

○ Normal weight: BMI 18.5 to 24.9

○ Overweight: BMI 25 to 29.9

○ Obesity (Class I): BMI 30 to 34.9

○ Obesity (Class II): BMI 35 to 39.9

○ Obesity (Class III): BMI 40 or greater

2. **Glasgow Coma Scale (GCS):** Scoring system for assessing consciousness and neurological status.

3. **Mini-Mental State Examination (MMSE):** A cognitive assessment tool to screen for cognitive impairment.

4. **Pain Scale:** Visual Analog Scale (VAS) or Numeric Rating Scale (NRS) for assessing pain intensity.

5. **Nutritional Assessment:** Use reference values for macronutrients, vitamins, and minerals.

6. **Pregnancy:**

○ Average pregnancy weight gain varies by trimester.

○ Fetal heart rate (FHR) reference ranges by gestational age.

7. **Pediatric Growth Charts:** Growth charts for children's height, weight, and head circumference.

Ensure that the reference charts you include in your book are up-to-date and relevant to the target audience. Additionally, consider guiding, interpreting and using these values in a clinical context.

Chapter Thirty-Six

References

Books:

1. Bates' Guide to Physical Examination and History Taking by Lynn S. Bickley MD FACP.

2. Clinical Examination: A Systematic Guide to Physical Diagnosis by Nicholas J. Talley and Simon O'Connor.

3. Seidel's Guide to Physical Examination by Jane W. Ball, Joyce E. Dains, and John A. Flynn.

4. Swartz's Textbook of Physical Diagnosis: History and Examination by Charles S. Swartz.

Medical Journals and Articles:

1. Epstein, R. M., & Hundert, E. M. (2002). Defining and assessing professional competence. JAMA, 287(2), 226-235.

2. Mangione, S. (1995). Cardiac auscultatory skills of physicians-in-training: a comparison of three English-speaking countries. The American Journal of Medicine, 98(1), 26-40.

3. Beck, R. S., Daughtridge, R., & Sloane, P. D. (2002). Physician-patient communication in the primary care office: a systematic review. The Journal of the American Board of Family Practice, 15(1), 25-38.

Websites and Online Resources:

1. Stanford Medicine 25: A valuable resource for physical examination techniques and teaching. Stanford Medicine 25

2. National Institutes of Health (NIH) Clinical Center: Offers educational resources on physical examination and clinical skills. NIH Clinical Center

Clinical Guidelines and Recommendations:

1. The American College of Physicians (ACP) - Clinical Guidelines for Physical Examination.

2. The U.S. Preventive Services Task Force (USPSTF) - Recommendations on various aspects of preventive health services and screenings.

Educational Institutions and Organizations:

1. Harvard Medical School - Provides educational resources and videos on physical examination techniques.

2. American Academy of Family Physicians (AAFP) - Offers educational materials and resources for family medicine practitioners.

Remember to properly cite and attribute these references in your book, adhering to your chosen citation style. These sources should help provide a strong foundation of evidence-based information and guidance for your readers interested in physical examination and history-taking.